The Dana Sourcebook of Brain Science

Resources for Teachers and Students

Fourth Edition

David Balog, Editor

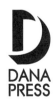

DANA PRESS   New York • Washington, D.C.

DANA
PRESS

The Dana Foundation
745 Fifth Avenue, Suite 900
New York, NY 10151

900 15th Street, NW
Washington, DC 20005

This publication is provided by the Dana Foundation free to participating schools. The Dana Foundation is a private philanthropic organization with particular interests in science, health, and education.

Please note: Additional copies or classroom sets may be ordered through www.dana.org. Also, access the online edition at www.dana.org.

ISBN 10: 1-932594-19-1
ISBN 13: 978-1-932594-19-5

LIBRARY OF CONGRESS CATALOGING-IN-PUBLICATION DATA
The Dana sourcebook of brain science : resources for secondary and post-secondary teachers and students / David Balog, editor.— 4th ed.
    p. cm.
  Includes bibliographical references and index.
  ISBN 1-932594-19-1 (alk. paper)
  1. Brain. I. Balog, David, 1957-
  QP376.D36 2006
  612.8'2—dc22   2006007158

A Dana Press publication
Jane Nevins, Editor in Chief

Contents

Preface

Lynn Wecker, Ph.D.,
Scientific Consultant, *The Dana Sourcebook*
of Brain Science, Fourth Edition

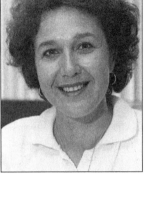

Because of new and improved brain research techniques, neuroscientists, neurologists, psychiatrists, and neurosurgeons are learning more every day about what has been called the most complex structure in the known universe—the human brain. We are steadily gaining understanding about how the brain functions, thinks, feels, imagines, and remembers.

Much of who we are and how we live depends on maintaining a healthy, active brain. Modern medicine is bringing new hope in the form of treatments for those whose brain has been compromised by disease or trauma.

The Dana Sourcebook of Brain Science: Resources for Teachers and Students is designed to introduce readers to brain science, its history, our current understanding of this complex system, and future directions. We are confident that you will find this book, our fourth edition, both informative and useful.

Scientific Lives

Part One:
A Life of Research, Advancing Our Knowledge of How the Brain Works

Editor's note: One way to study the brain is to become a researcher, conducting experiments, analyzing data, publishing results, and teaching. A leading scientist and researcher on depression and mental health, Huda Akil, Ph.D., is Gardner Quarton Distinguished University Professor of Neuroscience and Psychiatry and co-director of the Mental Health Research Institute at the University of Michigan. Dr. Akil is former president of the Society for Neuroscience, the world's largest organization of scientists devoted to the study of the brain.

Huda Akil, Ph.D.
A Leader in Emotions Research and an Advocate for Neuroscience Education

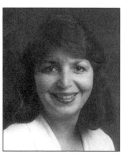

Huda Akil, Ph.D.

Dr. Huda Akil is a national advocate for the inclusion of neuroscience education in schools. She knows firsthand from teaching school-age children and adolescents that the brain fascinates them. "Young people are intensely interested in how their minds function and change as they develop. First-graders have asked me: 'What happens in our brains when we dream?' 'Where do the memories go when we forget?' Older students have profound questions about emotions, psychoactive drugs, brain-related illnesses, consciousness—in short all the questions that occupy neuroscientists. Sometimes these questions are intellectual or philosophical, but often they are intensely personal. After some of my high-school talks, students have asked me about friends who had died of suicide, family members suffering from Alzheimer's, classmates addicted to drugs, and other topics."

Dr. Akil describes her own love of science as a great gift. She was about twelve and living in her native city of Damascus, Syria, when the French nun who ran the library suggested that she read a book on the life of Marie Curie, who pioneered the therapeutic uses of radium early in the 20th century. "I was fascinated by both what she discovered and the fact that a young woman from a remote place could become so successful. I began to read everything I could on scientific discovery."

For young women today, Dr. Akil says there are excellent opportunities for pursuing scientific careers. "They typically demonstrate a great deal of talent and dedication. I do feel, however, that the career paths of men and women scientists are somewhat different, in that women peak a bit later, possibly because of the demands of child bearing and rearing. I hope that young women keep this in mind as they assess their careers and that institutions bear it in mind in their evaluations and willingness to support women."

In her study of depression, Dr. Akil thinks many genes likely interact to produce a vulnerability to an illness and none of these genes need be abnormal. Rather, combinations of variants of genes can result in different likelihoods of being prone or resistant to a given disorder. And, of course, the impact of the environment is critical. Says Dr. Akil, "Understanding emotionality is extremely challenging. It embodies the problems and the excitement of neuroscience." ■

Part Two:
Treating Patients With
Brain Diseases and Disorders

Editor's note: In addition to conducting research and teaching, brain scientists can also be "hands-on" doctors and surgeons. Benjamin S. Carson, Sr., M.D., one of the world's leading neurosurgeons, is director of pediatric neurosurgery at Johns Hopkins Medical Institutions. He is professor of neurosurgery, oncology, plastic surgery, and pediatrics at the Johns Hopkins University School of Medicine.

Benjamin S. Carson, Sr., M.D.
A Brain Surgeon Talks About
"Second Chances"

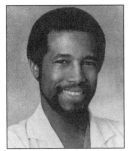

Benjamin Carson, M.D.

Not long ago, doctors whose practices focused on the brain had few tools to intervene significantly in their patients' lives. That has changed quickly. Brain doctors are now aggressively treating patients for stroke, seizures, acute trauma, psychoses, addiction, and even some neurodegenerative disorders.

One of these pioneers is Dr. Benjamin Carson. During his career he has gained international distinction for successful, delicate high-risk surgeries such as hemispherectomies—removing one side of the brain to treat those suffering from otherwise untreatable severe multiple seizures.

Dr. Carson speaks often to young students and emphasizes his own transition from poor inner-city kid in Detroit with failing grades to one of the most prestigious positions at one of the world's most renowned medical institutions. "Is it ever too late if you miss the boat the first time around? Well, I

have to tell you, when I was a youngster, many people would have said it was too late for me. No one certainly would have thought that I was going to grow up to be a physician."

His mother, Sonya, was determined to help, and she ordered Ben and his brother Curtis to read two books each week, which she, with only a third-grade education, pretended to review. "Once my mother made us start reading, what a tremendous change took place," says Dr. Carson.

Becoming a successful student didn't protect him from racist treatment, nor from his rage against it. In high school, a teacher scolded Ben's white classmates for letting a black student win the outstanding-achievement award. Then one day, Ben tried to stab a student who had changed the station on a radio. The student had a large metal belt buckle and the knife blade struck it and broke. Frightened by his anger, Ben ran home and prayed for hours. Devoutly religious like his mother, he says he has not lost his temper since.

Dr. Carson went on to win a college scholarship. "Later, I bombed out of my first set of comprehensive medical exams. The counselor suggested that there were a lot of things I could do besides medicine."

Dr. Carson at that point thought back to his mother's earlier encouragement to read. "I decided to concentrate on reading, which then made medical school a snap. Taking advantage of how we learn is incredibly important."

Dr. Carson believes in today's students. He is president and co-founder of the Carson Scholars Fund, which recognizes young people of all backgrounds for exceptional academic and humanitarian accomplishments. He says, "We need to start putting our resources where it counts and honoring our academic superstars." ■

Chapter 1

Revealing the Workings, the Wonder, of the Human Brain

Do each of the following, in succession. (<u>This is not a test</u>):

1. Visualize a place you'd like to be. Maybe it's lounging on a sunny summer day at the beach. Maybe it's in your living room, watching a favorite movie. Create the image of that place in your mind, and hold it for a minute or two.

2. Listen to the sounds in the room around you. Really listen. What do you hear? Low voices in conversation? Muffled laughter in the hall? Phones and computers ringing and beeping? See how many sounds you can differentiate.

3. Silently tap your fingers on the desk, one tap, one finger at a time, in succession. Then reverse the order of tapping. Then tap each finger twice, in succession; then in reverse.
Then three times....

4. Starting at 100, count backward by 7s.

5. Remember some event from your past. The first time you rode a bike all by yourself; your grandmother baking your favorite cookies; the first time you kissed someone other than a relative. Put yourself back in that place, and recall everything you can about it: Who was there with you? What were you wearing? What emotions were you feeling?

6. Now pinch yourself. Pick a tender spot on the inside of your elbow, and pinch the skin just hard enough to feel pain.

In performing these six tasks, you've just activated a good portion of your brain. Even something as "simple" as tapping your fingers in succession requires a phenomenal act of coordination among millions of nerve cells throughout the brain, all acting together in perfect timing to produce the signals that command your fingers to move.

If you had been lying inside a *PET* or *fMRI* scanner—tools of modern *neuroscience* that enable scientists to take images of the living brain as it works—the scans would show distinct areas of your brain "lighting up" as you did each task. Tapping your fingers in succession would activate groups of *neurons* in at least four distinct areas of the brain: the *prefrontal cortex,* where your brain makes the conscious decision to do the task; the *premotor cortex*, where you formulate the instructions for doing the task; the *motor cortex,* a sort of relay station that sends those instructions on to the arm and hand muscles that move the fingers; and the *cerebellum,* which supervises the whole process and adjusts your actions as necessary in response to external cues, such as where your hand is in relation to the desk. All of this takes place in a mere fraction of a second. Not such a "simple" task after all, from the brain's perspective.

Task number one, visual imagery, lights up the *visual cortex* in the back of the brain, as well as pathways leading to it from the eyes, along the optic nerve. Differentiating individual sounds around you activates the *auditory cortex* and associated areas. Tapping your fingers stimulates your motor cortex, which is involved in movement and muscle coordination. Counting backward by 7s is a complex *cognitive* task, and it calls upon the brain's center for higher thoughts in the prefrontal cortex.

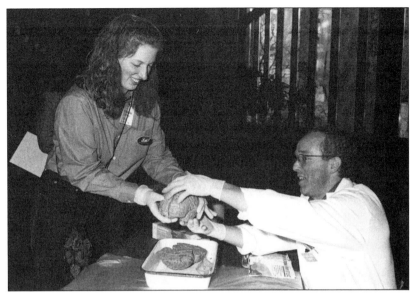

The brain, weighing approximately three pounds, makes us distinctively human. It encases 100 billion or more nerve cells and can send signals to thousands of other cells at a rate of about 200 miles an hour.

Recalling a *memory* from your past will likely activate the *hippocampus*, an inner-brain structure involved in memory, as well as other areas of the brain that correspond to the type of memory. For example, remembering the first time you rode a bike, a motor task, will light up the motor area of the brain; recalling the smell of Grandma's cookies would activate the *olfactory* center.

Lastly, when you pinched yourself, *pain receptors* in the nerves of the skin sent signals back to the brain to alert it to the location and intensity of the pain and to initiate corrective action if necessary (i.e., stop pinching!). If the pain was intense, the brain might release *endorphins,* natural *hormones* that block the transmission of pain signals. *Narcotic* drugs such as morphine imitate the action of these natural endorphins to fight pain.

The Most Complex Achievement of Nature

You've just taken a brief tour of your brain. It has taken scientists hundreds of years to figure out the bits of information you've just learned in a few minutes. If that seems like a long time for a

Note: Terms in italics are defined in "A Glossary of Key Brain Science Terms," beginning on page 99.

little bit of information, consider the complexity of the problem. The human brain is, as neuroscientist Joseph LeDoux, Ph.D., says in *The Emotional Brain,* "the most sophisticated machine imaginable, or unimaginable." It is composed of more than 100 billion nerve cells, each of which forms as many as 10,000 connections with other neurons. A typical brain weighs about three pounds, just two percent of the total body weight of a 150-pound person. But the brain uses between 20 percent and 25 percent of the body's oxygen and a substantial amount of the calories we consume in the form of the blood sugar *glucose.* The brain is also a nonstop factory of *neurotransmitters* that are critical to every thought and feeling we experience. About half of the 30,000 or so *genes* in the human *genome* are committed to building and operating the *central nervous system* (the brain and *spinal cord*).

tem result in more hospitalizations than any other disease group, including heart disease and cancer. Brain damage by stroke, they report, is one of the three greatest medical sources of death, depression causes the greatest disability for adults under the age of 45, and suicides continue to outnumber homicides by almost two to one. The aging of our population makes Alzheimer's and other *neurodegenerative diseases* an increasing public health concern. At the beginning of the lifespan, autism and related disorders have now been estimated at 1 in 166 births, roughly a tenfold increase in the past decade.

Evolution of the Brain

The modern human brain is the product of millennia of "evolutionary tinkering," says Dr. LeDoux. To figure out how it works, we need to "pick the brain apart in the hope that we will see what evo-

---

About half of the 30,000 or so genes in the human genome are committed to building the central nervous system (the brain and spinal cord).

In the process of deciphering the genetic code that is written in our *DNA*, learning the "blueprint" of our bodies is also likely to pave the way for a better understanding of the brain-based disorders and diseases that plague mankind and open new avenues for treating these disorders. This is an undertaking with enormous implications, because more than 60 million Americans are afflicted with a brain disorder—conditions that range from learning disabilities to *depression* to traumatic brain injury. That's nearly one in five of us. Look around you. If there are 25 students in your class, statistically 5 of you will be personally affected. Every one of us will personally know or care for someone who is affected by a brain disease or disorder.

Today, leading brain researchers report that the more than 1,000 disorders of the nervous sys-

lution was up to when it put the device together."

For centuries, "picking the brain apart" was, literally, how scientists learned how the brain worked. Actually, they usually picked apart the brains of other animals for clues as to how the human brain worked. As it turns out, the human brain is remarkably similar to the brains of other mammals, from rats right up to our closest cousins in the evolutionary tree, the great apes. In evolutionary terms, most of the structures in our brain are, in fact, primitive—that is, they have existed in much the same form for eons. These include the parts of the brain that control functions basic to survival, such as breathing, heart rate, and digestion. Such functions are centralized in the *brain stem,* located in the base of the brain, where the spinal cord meets the brain.

(continued on page 12)

Brain Imaging: A Closer Look

Computer technology has opened a window on the living brain. Before the early 1970s, only neuro-surgeons had seen a living human brain. Rapid advances in computer-generated imaging have allowed brain scientists and doctors to go inside the head and examine the structure and function of the brain in the living patient. Advances in the next few decades are expected to allow scientists to investigate how brain circuits work, how one part of the brain modifies the functions of other parts, and how these circuits adapt to new situations or damage to existing circuits. ■

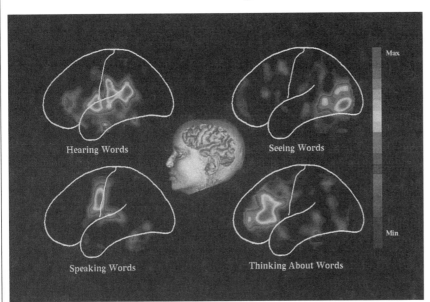

Measuring metabolism, *positron emission tomography,* or PET, allows scientists to recreate images of the living, functioning human brain. These images demonstrate that certain areas of the brain activate as the brain performs specific language tasks.

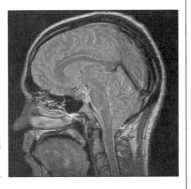

Magnetic resonance imaging, or MRI, employs powerful magnets to produce sharp, anatomical, three-dimensional images of the brain and all other parts of the body. In just one example of their use, neurosurgeons employ MRIs of the brain to plan surgery for epilepsy patients.

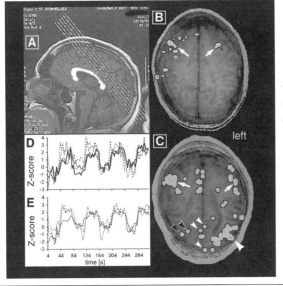

Expanding on conventional MRI by detecting variations in the response of hydrogen atoms when oxygen is present in the blood, *functional magnetic resonance imaging,* or fMRI, creates images that show which areas of the brain are working during specific tasks, behaviors, or thoughts. Here, image B represents the brain areas at work in a sighted person reading a one-syllable word in Braille. In image C, a visually-disabled person reads the same word in Braille and shows brain activity in additional areas—suggesting that the brain of the visually impaired person has reorganized its sensory pathways. (The graphs represented by D and E plot the data of the experiment.)

(continued from p. 10)

What Makes Human Brains So Special?

Clearly, humans have so-called specialized functions that rats, or even great apes, do not. So what makes humans so special? The key seems to lie in the prefrontal cortex, the forward-most section of the *cerebral cortex*, which is the brain's outermost layer of *gray matter*. This is the brain's command and control center, where higher cognitive functions are centralized, including the abilities for thinking, reasoning, believing, planning, and social *consciousness*—things that set us apart from other animals. The prefrontal cortex is more highly developed in humans than in any other primate, and it may not even exist in other mammals. (This is an area of continuing scientific exploration.)

In addition to examining the brains of other animals, scientists have made great strides in understanding brain function by observing people who have suffered trauma to the brain. Some of the most important breakthroughs in the biology of memory systems in the brain, for example, came from the study of a young man known as H.M., who underwent a radical surgery in which large sections of his *temporal lobes* were removed to control epileptic seizures. The surgery worked, but it left H.M. with a severe memory disorder in which he could learn, but not retain new information— he couldn't recall having met someone moments after that person had left the room. By observing H.M.'s behavior, and correlating it to the missing parts of his brain, scientists were able to learn which parts of the brain were responsible for certain behaviors. His case single-handedly shaped the course of memory research for decades.

While H.M. and legions of other brain-injury survivors spurred important advances in understanding the brain, for much of scientific history the brain was a black box, a mystery so profound it was long considered to be the realm of philosophy or religion, not science. The 15th-century philosopher René Descartes promoted the idea that the "mind" was separate from the brain or body—an idea that has stubbornly persisted even in this age of modern medicine, argues Antonio Damasio, M.D., Ph.D., in *Descartes' Error*. Indeed, medical science has only recently begun to recognize the links between psychological phenomena and physical health, or the power of the mind to influence healing in the body.

The drive to understand the brain's mysteries picked up speed as scientific methods advanced. As the 19th century ended, two scientists—an Italian physician named Camillo Golgi and a Spanish anatomist named Santiago Ramón y Cajal—forever changed our understanding of the brain and shared the 1906 Nobel Prize in Physiology or Medicine for their work. While Golgi's theories about brain function were later disproved, his techniques, in which he stained brain tissue with silver nitrate and other substances to reveal its inner structure, are still used today. Just as important, Golgi "opened scientists' eyes to the true complexity of the human brain," notes Bruce S. McEwen, Ph.D., a leading neuroscientist at Rockefeller University. Golgi, they say, was the

Scientists study the brains of other mammals to understand structures that bear remarkable similarity to the human brain, particularly those located in the brain stem.

first to see the brain as a network of connected cells. Even though he was wrong about how the cells were connected, his work spurred others, including Cajal, to look at the brain differently. Cajal advanced what later became known as "the neuron theory," which proposed that nerve cells were not structurally connected, as Golgi thought, but were separate cells connected in some other, unknown way.

Chemical, Electrical Pulses Spark Brain Cell Communication

Over the next couple of decades, scientists began to tease out the details of nerve cell communication. They learned that the connections Cajal had hypothesized to be the underpinnings of all human behavior were actually formed through a complex chemical signaling process. In this relay race of life, they learned, one cell squirts out a neurotransmitter, a chemical messenger, that crosses the *synaptic* gap between nerve cells and latches onto *receptors* on the surface of a neighboring cell. It wasn't long before dozens of neurotransmitters were discovered and systematically analyzed to determine their roles in cognition, behavior, and disease processes.

By the 1970s, it had become clear that brain function was the result of a complex interplay of chemical transmitters jolted into action by electrical impulses. The pulses were generated by ion channels within the neuron, which acted like the starting gun for the relay race of *interneuronal* communication. Today, scientists continue to elaborate the processes of cell-to-cell communication in exquisite detail, and a new arm of science has evolved that is now exploring the events that occur "beyond the receptor" within the *postsynaptic cell.*

The 1970s and 1980s were important decades for brain science. The development of PET (positron emission tomography) during this period enabled scientists to capture anatomical images of the living, functioning human brain and to begin to inventory the neurotransmitters involved in various behaviors or brain disorders. PET takes advantage of the fact that nerve cells *metabolize* the sugar glucose to derive the energy needed to perform their roles in brain function. By measuring changes in glucose uptake by nerve cells, PET enables scientists to determine which areas of the brain are activated during specific tasks (such as the finger-tapping exercise discussed earlier).

The introduction of PET got people thinking about other strategies for mapping the brain, and *MRI (magnetic resonance imaging)* soon followed. Rather than measuring how much glucose cells metabolize, MRI uses intensely powerful magnets and radio-wave pulses to capture images of the brain's structure (standard MRI) and function (fMRI). Standard MRI relies on the fact that molecules within cells, when placed in the strong magnetic field of an MRI scanner, "line up" in a certain fashion, much like the needle on a compass lines up with the Earth's magnetic field. When pulses of radio waves are applied to tissues with such alignment, the nuclei of individual molecules resonate the signals back in varying patterns that correspond to the chemical makeup of each area of tissue being studied. Scientists can then reconstruct anatomical images based on the patterns of resonance.

In recent years, sophisticated computer techniques have enabled brain imagers to take MRI to the next level, creating images that depict brain function in addition to anatomical structure. Using a standard MRI scanner, scientists can track which areas of the brain are active. When a specific region of the brain is active, neurons in that area use more oxygen. fMRI takes advantage of the different magnetic properties of oxygenated and deoxygenated blood, blood that has not been used by brain cells and blood that has been used. The relative concentrations of oxygenated and deoxygenated blood are measured and charted onto standard MR images of the brain to show which areas are "working."

Brain Function: The Sum of Many Parts

Imaging techniques such as PET and fMRI have revolutionized the field of brain science, enabling

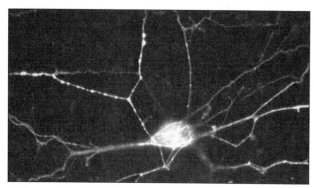

Here is an image of a single neuron taken from a rat brain, isolated in culture. Scientists estimate that the human brain has more than 100 billion neurons and about one quadrillion (one with 15 zeros) connections between neurons.

the precise mapping of brain functions and structures and permitting scientists to search out the roots of brain disorders or injuries. In addition, they have helped advance a "systems" view of brain function. According to this view, no one structure or area of the brain acts alone to drive a specific behavior or mental task. While certain brain areas may be specialized for certain tasks, brain function relies on networks of interconnected neurons. These specialized pathways enable the brain to analyze and assimilate information from external (e.g., sensory) as well as internal (e.g., hormonal) cues in order to respond with appropriate physical and psychological behaviors.

Systems neuroscience helps explain how people such as victims of stroke or head trauma, whose brains have been injured in a discrete site, can, over time, redevelop the functions lost as a result of the injury. Nerve cells in their brains in effect forge new pathways, bypassing the injured site and forming new connections, as if finding a new route to get to work after discovering that a bridge is out on the usual route. This ability to adapt, which scientists call *plasticity*, seems to be particularly strong in young brains, but "old" brains routinely learn new tricks, scientists have found.

Plasticity, in fact, plays a critical role in the entire life cycle of the brain, from its development in infancy, to its continual reshaping as learning occurs, to its ability to adapt to age-related changes that can lead to mental deterioration in later life. Now, new evidence suggests the brain may be even more plastic than previously thought. Turning one of the oldest tenets of neuroscience on its head, scientists recently discovered that nerve cells can regenerate, making the idea of brain repair following trauma or disease thinkable. Revealed at the end of the 20th century, this scientific breakthrough is sure to influence brain science for at least the next century.

Constructing the World's Most Sophisticated Machine

There is perhaps no time in the human life cycle during which plasticity is more important than in the period of nervous system development. A newborn baby's brain, scientists have learned, is not just a miniature version of an adult's. Instead, it is a work in progress, the world's most sophisticated machine in construction phase. Like the scaffolding that shapes the framework of a building, an initial framework of interneuronal "wiring" is present at birth, pre-set by nature via the genetic blueprints provided by the mother and father. The materials are also there: babies are born with virtually all of their lifetime store of nerve cells. (See developments in *stem cell research*, p. 23.) What remains is the "finish work" of the brain's communications architecture, the fine-tuning of a *quadrillion* cell-to-cell connections.

In humans, the fine-tuning phase unfolds over several developmental years. *"Nurture"* largely directs the completion of the wiring process, literally shaping the structure of the brain according to a child's early sensory experiences. During critical periods (or stages) of brain development, these early experiences stimulate neural activity in certain synaptic connections, which in turn become stronger and thrive. A "pruning" process ruled by a philosophy of "use it or lose it" ensues, during which synapses that are not routinely stimulated may wither and die. Within that period, "windows" of opportunity, during which the brain may be specially "primed" for learning certain skills such as language, open according to the developmental schedule of the brain regions underlying those skills. Since it's well known that humans can continue to learn and modify behavior throughout life, it's clear that the windows never really slam shut, even though they may become a bit sticky.

Children who fail to get the stimulation they need for proper brain development can become tragedies. In the 1990s, studies of Romanian orphans whose cries for comfort were never

oped. The prefrontal cortex, for example—the brain's center for reason, advance planning, and other higher functions—does not reach maturity until the early 20s. Since this part of the brain seems to act as a kind of cerebral "brake" to halt inappropriate or risky behaviors, some scientists believe sluggish development may explain difficulties in resisting impulsive behavior that some adolescents exhibit at times. The brain also has ultimate control over the ebb and flow of powerful hormones such as *adrenaline*, testosterone, and

> Numerous studies have also shown that babies who are held and caressed regularly do better developmentally and may reap the benefits throughout life.

answered or whose smiles were never encouraged, found lingering impairments in the children's basic social and thinking abilities and in their physical development. Numerous studies have also shown that babies who are held and caressed regularly do better developmentally and may reap the benefits throughout life.

The first few years of life are especially important, as they are periods of rapid change in the synapses. But new understandings about the developing brain indicate that the process of fine-tuning connections among neurons continues, to varying degrees, into adolescence. In fact, "brain development" probably never really ends—older adults are also capable of forming new synaptic connections and do when they learn new things. But the rapid-paced period during which external stimuli are critical to "normal" brain-building generally begins to dwindle around the mid-teen years.

Growing Pains in the Teenage Brain

Adolescence marks a turning point of sorts for the brain, as some of its structures are nearing maturity, while others are not yet fully devel-

estrogen, which themselves play critical roles in the changing adolescent body.

The teenage brain is also struggling to adapt to a shift in the circadian rhythm, the brain's internal biological clock, which drives the sleep-wake cycle. The secretion of *melatonin* sets the timing for this internal clock, a hormone the brain produces in response to the daily onset of darkness. In one study, researchers found that the further along in puberty teens were, the later at night their melatonin was secreted. In practice, that means teens' natural biological clock is telling them to go to sleep later, and to stay asleep longer.

The Aging Brain: Attitude Counts!

While the teenage brain faces its share of challenges as it weathers the storm of adolescence, aging undoubtedly poses the greatest challenge to the normal life cycle of the brain. But contrary to popular belief, the slow march of mental decline many people associate with aging is not inevitable. While many people do experience memory lapses as they age, even as early as their

40s, this too is not preordained. Scientists who study the aging brain have identified an intriguing set of circumstances and personal attributes that seem to protect some people from the age-related declines in mental ability that so many aging Americans fear. In fact, brain research is turning up a surprising amount of evidence that, when it comes to maintaining mental sharpness into old age, attitude counts.

Marilyn Albert, Ph.D., a neuropsychologist at Johns Hopkins University School of Medicine, and her colleagues have been following a large group of "high-functioning" elderly people in an effort to determine what specific attributes tend to characterize people who maintain high levels of mental abilities into their 70s and beyond. Moderate to strenuous physical activity and higher levels of formal education have been found to be key predictors of cognitive maintenance. But perhaps the most surprising correlate with successful aging is a psychosocial factor that scientists call "self-efficacy."

Dr. Albert defines self-efficacy as "the feeling that what you do makes a difference in the things that happen to you every day. It boils down to feelings of control." Scientists have theorized that our self-efficacy beliefs influence the types of activities we pursue, as well as how much effort we put into them, and how persistent we are if the task proves difficult. If we have doubts about our ability to accomplish something, we may be less likely to try it, or may give up more easily. A cycle ensues: If we fail to engage in challenging activities, our risk for cognitive decline increases as we age. We might be anxious or stressed about what we can no longer do, which sets off a cascade of stress hormones that can themselves contribute to memory lapses, and may damage brain systems in other ways as well. Scientists say that taking steps to assert control over one's life and surroundings, even in seemingly small ways, may help us to maintain our mental faculties well into old age.

According to Dr. Albert, specific activities that may help maintain memory and cognitive function in elderly people include mental exercises like word puzzles and games as well as physical excercises like walking long distances, climbing stairs, and lifting objects. Social stimulation appears to be important, too. Controlling weight, lowering cholesterol, and avoiding smoking are all associated with less disease of the blood vessels of both the heart and the brain.

Genetics and Stem-Cell Research: Breathtaking Vistas on the Great Biological Frontier

With all the advances neuroscience has seen in the past decades, the future holds even greater promise. New techniques in cellular, molecular, and genetic biology are opening up vast opportunities for scientists to explore.

Two major scientific accomplishments have recently focused public attention in these areas: the near complete sequencing and mapping of the human genome and discoveries related to stem cells, found in both human embryos and in adults.

The mapping and sequencing of the human genome, completed in 2003, is the crowning achievement of nearly two decades of effort by dozens of research laboratories. This identification of the makeup of the human genome basically provides the blueprint of the human body, with the 23 pairs of chromosomes and roughly 30,000 genes found in each of the approximately 100 trillion cells in the human body. Some researchers estimate that half of all human genes and the multiple proteins they produce play a role in developing and maintaining the central nervous system (the brain and spinal cord). (For a more in-depth look at genes and the brain, turn to p. 19.)

Having access to the human genome sequences will help brain researchers in four areas: helping brain medicine diagnose disease, determining genetic versus environmental effects, deciphering the underlying mechanisms of disease, and developing effective medications and treatments.

Our understanding of the role of human DNA increased even more just recently. Neuroscientist

Thomas Insel, Ph.D., of the National Institute of Mental Health, says, "The good news is that we have extraordinary new tools and technologies with which to address…urgent public health challenges." The Human Genome Project provided a consensus map of human DNA but it failed to describe variation. "Because variation is the key to understanding individual vulnerability and resistance to disease as well as human diversity, a map of human DNA variation may be even more informative than the original consensus map. [The year 2006] marks the completion of the 'HapMap' project, the first comprehensive map of human haplotypes."

types) when grown in culture and treated with appropriate inducing factors.

The potential use of such stem cells for the treatment of *neurodegenerative disorders* such as Parkinson's disease and to replace damaged neural tissue could provide a whole new dimension to research and ultimately to treatment of some of our most difficult brain diseases and disorders. (For a more in-depth look at stem cell research, turn to p. 23.)

As scientists learn more about cellular and genetic biology, they are discovering new keys that may unlock the mysteries of the devastating brain disorders that continue to ravage mankind.

The big advance will be to develop functional imaging techniques that show us—as it is happening— how various areas of the brain interact.

With the HapMap, scientists will begin to learn how genes vary in the population. The question of how individual variations in DNA sequences are associated with risks for diseases can now be answered not only for single gene disease (such as Huntington's disease) but also for complex genetic diseases that affect the brain and the nervous system.

Another major development in cellular biology has come in discoveries related to stem cells. Stem cells are "blank," undifferentiated cells that can grow into heart cells, kidney cells, or other cells of the body. Originally thought to be found only in embryos, stem cells have unexpectedly been discovered in adult brains and other parts of the body.

In experiments, researchers have shown that stem cells can be transplanted into various regions of the brain, where they develop into both neurons and *glia*. Moreover, researchers now believe that other types of stem cells—from bone marrow, muscle, or skin—can be made to differentiate into neurons (and even neurons of specific

A large group of leading brain scientists from around the world has outlined specific areas of neuroscience in which rapid advances are forecast. Already, progress has been made in each of these areas. True breakthroughs that will change the way we think about the brain and its disorders are imminent.

With great knowledge in neuroscience comes great responsibility. The emerging field of *neuroethics* has begun to focus on the ethical implications of our increased ability to understand and change the brain. Neuroscientists are joining with other scientists, other professionals, and concerned citizens to consider how this power can best be used for the greatest public good.

Neurologist Guy M. McKhann, M.D., of Johns Hopkins University, predicts great advances in the next few decades in imaging, which actually now does not take place in real time with brain activity—that is, the images show brain systems' activity milliseconds after it begins. "The big advance," he says, "will be to develop functional imaging techniques that show us—as it is happening—how various areas of the brain interact. That is, we will see not only the location of brain activity but also its speed. Whatever the method, this souped-up imaging will enable us to investigate how brain circuits work, how one part of the brain modifies the functions of other parts, and how these circuits adapt to new situations or damage to existing circuits."

Dr. McKhann also says that we will be able to use imaging to study cell transplants in the brain. "Transplanted cells and their changes can be tracked by molecules on their surfaces. Specific markers can be attached to those molecules as tags that can be spotted by imaging, like radio collars on wolves moved to a new terrain. Other cells, scavenger cells that are part of our immune system, can be tracked into and out of the brain as they respond to injury or to therapies."

Dr. Insel says that recent advances have enhanced our ability to visualize individual cells, even in the living brain. "In addition," he says, "both structural and functional studies of the whole brain have been enhanced to allow neuro-scientists to identify pathways for information in the brain. With imaging we can map the remarkable plasticity in the human cortex, the circuits for processing faces and language and even the evidence for information that is encoded without any conscious awareness. Marcus Raichle, M.D., a pioneer in *brain imaging,* says that "several issues are likely to be of increasing importance to our future understanding of human brain function and likely will receive increasing attention from the neuroimaging community. These include individual differences, development (brain maturation), and the activities of the "resting brain."

"I ask myself how many of the advances in the last 25 years of brain science I would have predicted," says Dr. McKhann. "Not many. Some came from logical, sequential explorations of how the brain works. Others were great leaps that kicked over strongly held beliefs. Others came through luck, albeit the luck of very patient and alert investigators. The same combination will shape the next 25 years of brain research." ■

Chapter 2

Genes and the Brain

Imagine a homework assignment in which you must read and understand the "Book of Life," a story with 3.3 billion letters. Printed out, the letters would fill a volume of books that would reach as high as the Washington Monument. Oh, and the letters are all either A, C, G, or T, arranged in seemingly endless combinations. Some of the "words" are millions of letters long, and you'll need to figure out where one ends and another begins. Then you'll need to find out what the words mean (there's no dictionary), and how they interplay with all the other words in the book.

That is essentially the task that was undertaken by the Human Genome Project, a government-funded effort to "read" the human genome, and a parallel effort by Celera Genomics, a private company. The genome contains the complete instruction manual for Homo sapiens, written in chemical code along the twisted *double-helix* strands of DNA that are carried within each of the 100 trillion cells in the human body (except in mature red blood cells).

The mapping and sequencing of the human genome, completed in 2003, culminates nearly five decades of investigation following the first description of the double-helix model of DNA by James D. Watson and Francis Crick in 1953. Watson and Crick's view of DNA successfully described how molecules of nucleic acid could not only carry tremendous amounts of information, but could also copy themselves accurately each time a cell divides.

With the mapping and sequencing of the human genome, for the first time scientists can see the entire landscape of all the human chromosomes and how the genes are organized on the chromosomes. Encoded in the twists of our DNA are about 30,000 genes, the critical "words" in the Book of Life. They determine every inherited trait we have, from the color of our eyes to the size of our feet, and possibly even behavioral traits such as an inclination to be aggressive or our desire for affection. More important, they tell us what diseases we may be susceptible to and those we may be protected from, as well as what medicines we might respond to in the event of illness.

In short, understanding the Book of Life has the potential to change everything about health, medicine, and life in general. Welcome to the Genomics Era.

Genomics will affect every field of medical science, but its significance to brain science is particularly great. As much as half of the genome's instruction manual—as many as 15,000 genes—is thought to be devoted to the workings of the central nervous system (the brain and spinal cord) and peripheral nerves. One surprise of the genome projects was that humans have only about twice as many genes as fruit flies and roundworms, two "simpler" species used as models for biological systems in science and medicine. Many of the "extra" genes in humans are thought to be devoted to the development,

(continued on page 22)

Basic Genetics—A Brief Guide

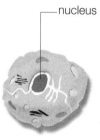

nucleus

A human cell

Each of the 100 trillion cells in the human body (except mature red blood cells) contains a copy of the entire human genome—all the genetic information necessary to build a human being. The cell nucleus is a separate compartment in the cell that contains six feet of DNA packed into 23 pairs of chromosomes. We each inherit one set of 23 chromosomes from our mother and another set from our father. Egg and sperm cells carry single sets of 23 chromosomes.

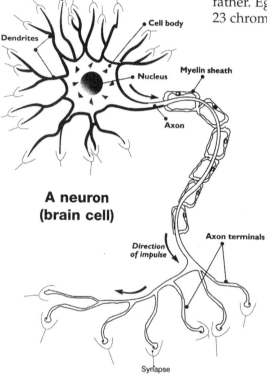

Synapse

Cell body

Dendrites

Nucleus

Myelin sheath

Axon

A neuron (brain cell)

Direction of impulse

Axon terminals

Synapse

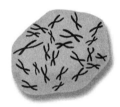

DNA

The material from which the 46 chromosomes in each cell's nucleus are formed is called DNA (*deoxyribonucleic acid*). DNA contains the codes for the body's approximately 30,000 genes, governing all aspects of cell growth and inheritance. DNA has a double-helix structure—two intertwined strands resembling a spiraling ladder. DNA consists of just a few kinds of atoms: carbon, hydrogen, oxygen, nitrogen, and phosphorus. Combinations of these atoms form the sugar-phosphate backbone of the DNA—the sides of the ladder.

A chromosome

In the nucleus of any normal human cell there are 23 sets of chromosomes. Within each of the 46 chromosomes is bundled a double-stranded helix of DNA. Each of the human chromosomes contains genes, the major functional units of DNA.

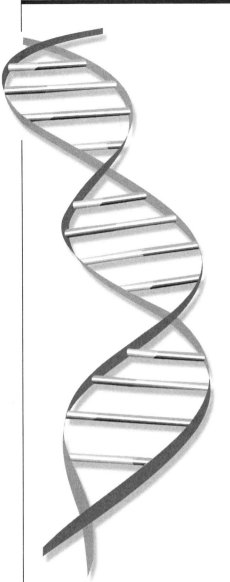

A gene

Each gene is a segment of DNA, typically several thousand base pairs long. Genes are copied into a molecule of *RNA (ribonucleic acid),* which is translated to make a specific molecule, usually an *amino acid.* Combinations of the atoms carbon, hydrogen, oxygen, nitrogen, and phosphorus form the four chemical bases in DNA: adenine (A), thymine (T), guanine (G), and cytosine (C). The bases form interlocking pairs that can fit together in only one way: A pairs with T; G pairs with C. Each such pair is called a base pair of DNA.

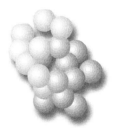

A protein

Proteins, which are made up of amino acids, are the body's workhorses, essential components of all organs and chemical activities. Their function depends on their shapes, which are determined by the roughly 30,000 genes in the cell nucleus.

Mutation

Mutations are changes in DNA spelling that can result in abnormal proteins that do not function normally and therefore cause health problems.

Three DNA bases are deleted in the mutated sequence below, resulting in the deletion of an *amino acid* (phenylalanine) from the CF protein. People with the abnormal protein develop cystic fibrosis.

Normal CF (cystic fibrosis) sequence

▽ ■ ■ ▲ ◆ ● ★
ATT ATC ATC TTT GGT GTT TCC

Mutated CF sequence

▽ ■   ▲ ◆ ● ★
ATT ATC   TTT GGT GTT TCC

SNP

Pronounced "snip," SNPs (single nucleotide polymorphisms) are one-letter variations in the DNA sequence. SNPs contribute to differences among individuals. The majority have no effect; others cause subtle differences in countless characteristics, such as appearance, while some affect the risk for certain diseases.

C G G T A C T T G A G G C T A Person 1
C G G T A C T C G A G G C T A Person 2

Sources:
National Human Genome Research Institute: (*www.nhgri.nih.gov*); Howard Hughes Medical Institute: *Blazing a Genetic Trail*, (*www.hhmi.org*); Public Broadcasting System, WGBH: *DNA Workshop* (*www.pbs.org/WGBH*); CNN: "Scientists Sequence First Human Chromosome," (*www.cnn.com*).

(continued from p. 19)
structure, and function of the brain—a testament to the complexity of the organ that most differentiates us from every other living thing on earth.

Not So Different from a Fruit Fly

Still, experts remind us that at the level of individual brain cells (neurons) we're not all that different from fruit flies. Many of the most basic mechanisms of brain function—how cells communicate with one another or how memories are processed, among others—are basically the same in humans and fruit flies, as well as in mice, chimpanzees, and other species. In the spirit of "if it's not broken, don't fix it," such processes have been conserved by the forces of evolution. Much of the human brain's complexity is more likely a result of our having so many more neurons interconnected in so many more ways. Think of it as your home PC versus a huge supercomputer: the basic operating systems are the same, but the supercomputer has far more processing power.

The sequencing of the human genome—and, more important, determining the function of all those genes—will reveal the brain's deepest secrets: why we act the way we do; why some things are easier to learn than others; how our brain develops from conception through adulthood, including the critical teenage years when the brain undergoes a dramatic "pruning" process to streamline its circuits. It will also give us new information about the genetic components of brain diseases, which include a wide array of disorders ranging from attention deficit disorder to Alzheimer's disease and mental illnesses such as depression and schizophrenia. Scientists have struggled for years to find the genes at the root of many of these brain disorders; with the sequence in hand, the searches will be much speedier.

Here's Your Genome

What does all this mean to you? Imagine a time in your future when you can visit a human genome laboratory and a week later, get back a DVD with your personal genome spelled out. It comes with an editorial describing your life story, as told by your genes. It tells you what illnesses for which you may be at risk and which *recessive* genes you may have that could be passed along to your children. Armed with information about your risk, you could take steps to protect yourself. These might include lifestyle changes that reduce the likelihood of your exposure to "triggers" in the environment that might set the disease process in motion, or taking medications genetically formulated to alter the function of the gene or genes that put you at risk.

Sound like a brave new world? With the knowledge of our genome, the potential for changing medicine for the better, and the world we live in, is tremendous. Moreover, a significant part of genetics research is being devoted to understanding the ethical, legal, and social implications of the sequencing effort and to finding ways to safeguard against abuses and ensure the privacy of individuals in the Genomics Era.

While the sequence of the human genome is now a matter of public information, the task before genomics scientists has merely begun. Now, the challenge is to create the "dictionary" that explains each word in the Book of Life: what it means, what roles it plays in development and biological function, and what goes wrong when disease or illness strikes. This phase will be the most difficult by far. When complete, everything we now know—about science, medicine, and life overall—will forever change. ■

Chapter 3

Stem Cells and Brain Research

By Fred H. Gage, Ph.D.

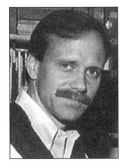

Fred H. Gage, Ph.D.

Dr. Gage is professor, the Laboratory of Genetics, at the Salk Institute for Biological Studies, La Jolla, CA. His current areas of specialization are regeneration and neurogenesis in the adult nervous system.

Almost every day a newspaper article, news magazine piece, or television news story extols the miraculous possibilities of replacing diseased organs with tissue made in the laboratory from stem cells or raises nightmarish specters of unregulated harvesting of stem cells to create clones. The interest in stem cell research recently reached such a fever pitch that when a Korean scientist fabricated claims to have generated new stem cell lines using nuclear transfer technology, the story was covered by the world press on a daily basis. Stem cell research does offer real promise and does raise real concerns, but unfortunately the public has not been adequately informed about the science behind the debate.

The hopes and promises for the use of these cells as therapies for devastating and currently untreatable diseases are being counterbalanced by the concerns over the ethical issues associated with the source of the cells. The discussion of stem cells also has been linked to discussions of cloning humans, as well as to the use of fetal tissue for transplantation. Trying to untangle unrelated issues and clarifying what is currently known versus what is believed to be true can help us make informed decisions. An informed public will make rational decisions about the use of stem cells and can provide knowledgeable support in advancing this potentially useful field of biomedical research.

So, What Is a Stem Cell?

In its simplest form, a stem cell is any cell that can divide and produce a cell like itself (self-renewal) and produce another progeny that gives rise to a mature cell of any organ of the body—that is, blood, brain, liver, and so on. Some stem cells are "totipotent" cells; that is, they can give rise to a fully developed organism. For instance, a fertilized egg has this potential for about four days. These cells can be produced through human reproduction or in the laboratory through in vitro fertilization (IVF), a life-giving procedure that helps infertile couples conceive a child.

Within about eight days after fertilization, the totipotent stem cell divides, matures, and gives rise to more restricted cells called "pluripotent" stem cells. These cells can self-renew and can give rise to any cell of the body. Pluripotent cells have, as far as we understand now, lost the potential to form an organ and certainly cannot form a fully developed organism. This complex cellular development takes place before organs begin to form in the embryo or even before the embryo leaves the fallopian tubes and implants in the uterus.

These more restricted pluripotent cells are called embryonic stem (ES) cells and are the focus of both the promise and concern currently being expressed at national and international levels.

The promise is based on the fact that these cells can divide indefinitely and may be able to be used to replace missing, damaged, or dying cells in any organ of the developing and adult body. Certain diseases, in which specific types of cells are damaged, as in diabetes, Parkinson's disease, heart disease, and cancers, are likely to be the first targets for such therapeutic applications.

A less well described, but more immediate use of human ES cells is as a tool to understand human disease. ES cells generated from humans with disease can be grown in culture indefinitely and induced to become any cell of the human body. Therefore, the cells can be used to study and discover how diseases begin and develop in human diseased cells. These same cells can then be used to screen drug libraries to find new therapeutic agents that are safe to "normal" human cells and that could prevent the development of the disease.

The concern about human cloning is a very different issue and is not supported or encouraged by the public, politicians, ethicists, or scientists. Human cloning would involve taking DNA from one person and putting it in a donor egg that has had its DNA removed. This newly engineered egg would then be implanted in a woman who would carry the resulting child to term. That child would have the same or similar DNA content as the person who originally donated the DNA. This is not only unacceptable on ethical grounds, but all animals that have been generated by this method have been shown to be sick or deformed in some way.

Where Can Stem Cells Be Obtained, and How Do Various Types of Stem Cells Differ?

Once an embryo implants in the uterus and begins to make specific organs, at about 25 days after fertilization, separate groups of more mature stem cells take up residence in the different organs (blood, skin, brain, etc.) and contribute to making the cells of each organ. These cells remain in the organ throughout life and can be obtained at any time in development as well as in adulthood, but are more abundant early during development, when the fetus is growing. These later cells are called organ-restricted, "multipotent" stem cells (sometimes referred to as adult stem cells, because a limited number remain in and can be isolated from adult organs).

Great interest and effort are being put into investigating both ES cells and multipotent stem cells, but it is not clear whether the multipotent (adult stem) cells live as long or are as viable as the pluripotent ES cells. Research shows that multipotent cells are certainly not as versatile or potent as ES cells.

Our knowledge is currently too limited for making a decision as to which cells will be the best or most efficacious for which therapy. However, it is quite likely that, through a careful comparison of ES cells and multipotent cells, a clearer understanding will emerge as to the best, safest, and most ethical way to use stem cells for the treatment of human diseases.

Pluripotent ES cells can be obtained from the surplus fertilized eggs produced by fertility clinics through IVF. Most of these surplus fertilized eggs are not used and are discarded. This fact contributed to the recent decision in the United Kingdom to approve financial support for the evaluation of new human embryonic cells to develop therapies for human disease. The United States approved a plan permitting the use of a limited number of existing ES cell lines in 2001.

In the United States, unregulated research continues to be carried out by private companies using private funding. In 2004 a ballot initiative was passed in California to support human stem cell research in that state by issuance of a bond. The funds are currently tied up in litigation, but planning for a new California Institute of Regenerative Medicine is under way to administer this statewide research effort.

While other states are beginning to follow California's lead, approval of federal support for the generation of new ES cells would guarantee that extensive guidelines could be enforced for federally funded research. Oversight of federally funded research would cover such issues as the source of cells, informed consent, and measures to ensure safety and the ethical use of ES cells.

It is important to remember that the information gained from research sponsored by federal funding is open to the public and available for scientists to use for their own studies and potential therapeutic applications.

The biomedical research community generally supports the study of ES cells for their potential value in understanding and treating a variety of diseases unresponsive to current therapies, but like most citizens of this country, the scientific community would support fully enforceable guidelines that would permit the best open and ethical information to be obtained. Only by obtaining accurate, responsible, and high-quality information can people make informed decisions and explain our positions to our local and national representatives. ■

Chapter 4
Advances in Brain Research

A Look at Remarkable Achievements and
Far-Reaching Goals in Specific Areas of
Brain Science and Brain Medicine

- Heredity ■ Neural Imaging ■ Learning ■ Neuroimmunology

- Neuroethics ■ Neurosurgery and Neurology ■ The Adolescent Brain

- Stroke, or Brain Attack ■ Stress ■ Alzheimer's Disease ■ Depression

- Memory ■ Emotions ■ The Developing Nervous System

- Spinal Cord Repair ■ Parkinson's Disease ■ Epilepsy

- Multiple Sclerosis ■ Brain Injury ■ Brain Tumor

- Pain ■ Addiction ■ Basic Brain Knowledge ■ Cell Replacement

- Neural Repair ■ Electronic Aids ■ Drug Discovery

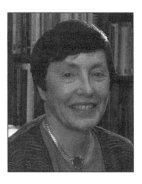

The Role of Nature: Innate Gifts and Hereditary Factors

By Nancy C. Andreasen, M.D., Ph.D.

Webster's New World Dictionary defines the word create as "to cause to come into existence; make; originate; to bring about; give rise to; cause." Nancy C. Andreasen, M.D., Ph.D., who began her career as a scholar in Renaissance literature and is now a world leader in the study and treatment of schizophrenia, has analyzed firsthand accounts of the creative process from some of the most accomplished artists and scientists in history—from da Vinci to Tchaikovsky to Neil Simon. Andreasen looks at creativity through many lenses: one's brain, one's genes, and one's environment. She asks questions about the nature of highly creative brains.

The environment into which an individual is born makes a difference. Had Leonardo or Michelangelo been born two hundred years earlier or later, we would never have had the body of work that they produced. Anatomical dissections would not have been possible at an earlier time. Patrons and prosperity would not have been there to support them. Without Lorenzo, Michelangelo would not have been a sculptor. Had Julius II not commissioned the Sistine ceiling, Michelangelo would not have turned his hand to fresco. Both Leonardo and Michelangelo would have had a "creative nature," but it might never have become manifest had they lacked the nurture of a supportive environment....

Environment makes a difference!...

But so does nature. "Nature" is related to heredity, but not identical.

Where does creative genius come from? How does it arise? These are both questions that everyone would like to answer.

Our case studies also shed light on these questions. Think about how the brains of Leonardo and Michelangelo were created.

When these two men were conceived, they were the consequence of shuffling the cards in the genetic deck, with half of the genes coming from the mother and half from the father. A grand challenge in modern science is to figure out how those shuffled genes become translated into complete living organisms, many of them complicated almost beyond imagination. A human being, for example, is somehow produced by forty-six chromosomes and about thirty thousand genes, give or take a few. Somehow these genes must orchestrate the creation of cells and their differentiation so that they form diverse body organs, such as the liver, the kidneys, and the brain. Within the brain there are also many different types of cells. But, most importantly, the human brain is defined by the multiple and complex ways that these cells are connected to one another. At this moment we still know very little about how genes affect the development of the brain in the uterus before birth, or during childhood, adolescence, and adult life. We are almost totally clueless about how genes become translated into complex human traits such as creativity or personality or cognitive style. Lots of people are studying the genetic regulation of small parts of the process. We know that genes produce proteins with funny names like MAP or GAP or SNAP, which affect components of brain development and maturation, such as neurogenesis or synapse formation. But we do not know much (yet) about how genes affect the interconnectedness of the trillions of neurons in our brains and the quadrillions of synapses that talk back and forth to one another. Thus we can say nothing at present about how genes, working at the molecular level, might have an influence on the creation of the creative brain. For now, we have to rely on speculations and hunches, combined with crude empirical methods, such as family studies of heritability.

What we perhaps can say is that Mother Nature gives creative people brains that are well designed for perceiving and thinking in original ways. Some of that influence must be coded in the genetic shuffle in ways that we do not yet understand. And very likely the gift given by Mother Nature is an enriched ability to make novel associations and to self-organize in the midst of apparent disorganization or even chaos.

The creative brain may appear unexpectedly, in people who simply seem to have been given innate gifts. Or it may appear within a hereditary context, in people who seem to have a genetic endowment that makes them creative.

(Excerpted from *The Creating Brain: The Neuroscience of Genius,* by Nancy C. Andreasen, M.D., Ph.D. Dana Press, Washington, DC, 2005.)

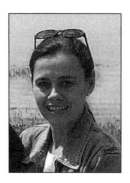

New Frontiers in Neural Imaging

By Brenda Patoine

The ability to view the living human brain began a revolution in brain research and brain medicine more than 30 years ago. Today, new technologies—and the ways in which neuroscientists are employing them—are driving advances beyond what any expert predicted. Sophisticated images and microscopy techniques are offering an increasingly clearer view of what is

happening below the surface of our skulls. Author Brenda Patoine is a freelance science and medical writer based in LaGrangeville, NY.

Today, sophisticated images from scans and new microscopy techniques are offering an unparalleled glimpse into our brains.

Some of the greatest excitement in neural imaging right now is coming from optical imaging, a technology that combines two-photon excitation microscopy with fluorescent dyes that label individual molecules in living tissue.

Two-photon microscopes use long wavelength light, supplied by lasers, to penetrate tissue more deeply and with less damage than other optical imaging tools. Critical to its innovation was the identification and cloning of the gene for green fluorescent protein (GFP) in 1994. GFP is a naturally occurring jellyfish protein that makes cell tissue forced to express it light up like a neon sign when viewed with this type of microscope.

A recent meeting on neural imaging at Cold Spring Harbor Laboratory in New York brought together a few dozen of the world's leading experts to compare notes, debate technical hurdles, and share some of the most remarkable video and still images of mammalian brains in action.

Among alternative methods, "there's no competition for optical imaging," says Karel Svoboda of Cold Spring Harbor, who co-chaired the meeting. "Using genetic tricks with GFP and its dozens of variants, you can now put into neurons fluorescent markers of structure, of specific molecules, or of cellular function. This has enabled a better understanding not only of the structural biology of the brain at the level of synaptic circuits, but also has begun to help us learn about the function of populations of neurons in the intact brain."

Grappling With Circuits

New imaging methods are also making a huge impact on systems neuroscience, which seeks to construct "wiring diagrams" that correlate brain activity to specific behaviors. While electrical recording studies can measure activity across synaptic connections, David Kleinfeld, a neuro-physicist at the University of California, San Diego, says optical imaging now makes it possible "to observe how different sensory and motor patterns sculpt and resculpt the connectivity." The ultimate goal is to use different types of GFP-based indicators in various types of neurons to understand how they interact and influence one another.

Birth of Modern Imaging

Computerized tomography (CT) marked the beginning of the modern era of neural imaging. "CT was a remarkable advance, because it was the first time you could look into the brain of a living person," says Arthur Toga, who heads the Laboratory of Neuro Imaging at the University of California, Los Angeles.

Next came magnetic resonance imaging (MRI), and later functional MRI (fMRI) as well as positron emission tomography (PET), which let us see patterns of brain activity that underlie mental functions and pathological states.

In terms of clinical practice, neuroimaging has undoubtedly had the greatest impact on neurosurgery. Brain scans are routinely used presurgically and increasingly during surgery to identify critical brain structures to be avoided and to guide the surgeon's scalpel to a tumor or vascular occlusion.

Imaging is also playing a greater role in neurology and psychiatry clinical practices. One sign of this progression is the government's recent announcement that Medicare will cover the cost of PET scans in certain people suspected of having Alzheimer's disease. Recently, the NIH launched a five-year, 50-site study designed to identify biological markers for Alzheimer's through brain imaging, with the ultimate goal of improving early diagnosis and intervention.

Integration Is Key

The integration of varied disciplines from mathematics to computer science has been instrumental in allowing scientists literally to see the brain in a whole new way. Says Toga, "What's now occurring is the application of complex computational strategies that extract more information out of the images....we can take that data, 'massage' it, compare it against statistical and imaging databases, and apply a variety of visualization algorithms to look at it in new ways."

(Adapted from "Peering Into the Brain: New Frontiers in Neural Imaging," by Brenda Patoine, *BrainWork: The Neuroscience Newsletter*, Vol. 15, No. 4, July–August, 2005. Dana Press, Washington, DC.)

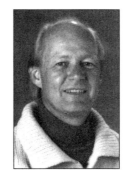 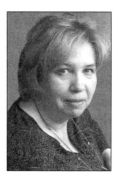

Listening to Learn

By Peter Perret and Janet Fox

Does music physically change the brain? Is music a primary language of the brain? Can music help young students with short attention spans, dyslexia, and other learning abilities? In a program organized by Peter Perret, 26-year director of the Winston-Salem Symphony, and described here with the help of writer Janet Fox, five musicians played for and interacted with first graders. More than two years after their visits, the children did strikingly better on state tests than the third-grade class that preceded them. The effect of the arts on the brain is one of the most intriguing areas of brain research.

Brain research indicates that new tasks and concepts are learned efficiently when instruction involves frequency, intensity, cross-training, and motivation and attention. That means the students must be exposed to the material over and over, that they must practice the new skills in a concentrated manner, that comprehension is enhanced when related skills and concepts are taught simultaneously, and that maintaining an interest in the material matters. Joaquin Fuster puts it this way (emphasis mine): *"Contiguity, repetition, and emotional load* seem to be the most decisive strengtheners of synaptic contact in the making of a cognitive network."

Musicians may not use the words *sequenced, cumulative, mutisensory, contiguous, repetitive,* and *emotionally loaded,* but these adjectives add up to a pretty good description of their own musical education and training. Musicians know from experience that music is best taught in an orderly sequence, and that new information is learned most easily when it builds on what has been previously presented and learned. That's exactly the way their musical training proceeds; it is sequenced and cumulative. Musicians also know from their own training that none of the elements of a subject can be fully understood in isolation. They quite naturally combine many components and aspects of a topic in every lesson they teach. It's second nature to them to cluster and combine things that "go together," or that touch each other, and so they have a deep understanding of *contiguity....*

What musicians know is that practice doesn't make perfect but that *practice makes permanent.* That's why music teachers tend to be so picky about their students' posture, how they place their fingers, when they take breaths, and so forth. It doesn't take many repetitions to lock in a particular way of doing something, and an awkward, limiting way of getting the task done can be very difficult to unlearn, or to replace with a better technique. Music teachers, and dance teachers, too, often prefer to get students before they have had much or any training, because these students are less likely to have ingrained bad habits and faulty techniques.

And finally, there is "emotional load." No one needs scientific proof that we learn something more easily when the process is pleasant. For a musician, nothing is more enjoyable than playing

music. Our quintet members carry into the classroom a deep love of music. The music they play is at the very least a "pleasure technology," a time-honored way of lifting spirits and lightening tasks.

So what is going on with these third graders, lying on their stomachs, listening for images as the music washes over them, then writing down the associations and emotions suggested by the sounds? A sequenced pattern of sounds that is meaningful because the children probably came into the world with its grammar encoded in their brains. A set of instruments whose intermingled and commingled voices have been heard repeatedly over a period of weeks. An exercise that builds on the children's knowledge of the elements of music, starting with musical opposites. A task that requires them to connect something to something quite different, a sound to an internal state or remembered experience. A challenge to thought that is bathed in the pure pleasure of music masterfully played.

What is going on is learning.

(Excerpted from *A Well-Tempered Mind: Using Music to Help Children Listen and Learn,* by Peter Perret and Janet Fox. Dana Press, Washington, DC, 2004.)

Neuroimmunology: A Connection with the Brain

By Dan Gordon

Neuroimmunology, whose complex work focuses on the brain, the immune system, and their interactions, holds the potential for conquering ills as diverse as spinal cord injury, multiple sclerosis, and bodily reactions to pathogens, both naturally occurring and intentionally inflicted. Dan Gordon is Senior Editor at Dana Press and editor of The Dana Sourcebook of Immunology: Resources for Teachers and Students.

Immunology and neuroscience may well be the two most complex fields of biomedical research today. Neuroimmunology, the study of the interaction between our central nervous system (the brain and spinal cord) and our immune system, melds these two disciplines.

Although questions about how your immune cells affect the brain and how your brain influences immune function are not new, neuroimmunology as a field of research is relatively young. The term has been in use only since the 1960s, and it was just 30 years ago that a neuroimmunology branch was established at the National Institutes of Health, the federal agency responsible for advancing biomedical research. Today the study of nervous system—immune system interactions is thriving, as more and more scientists from diverse areas of medical research are drawn into the field.

Immune Privileged

Scientists have long understood that the brain, with its complex pathways of nerve connections developed over a lifetime of experiences, holds special status regarding how the immune system defends it. This "immune privilege" may be the brain's way of protecting its delicate tissue from potential damage by immune cells in their rush to eliminate a threat.

In their normal response, immune cells release biochemicals that neutralize foreign particles and signal other components of the immune system to react to the threat. Some of these chemicals are toxic to nerve cells and can damage or kill them, disrupting brain function. Inflammation, another weapon the immune system uses to eliminate its enemies, can quickly spiral out of control in the central nervous system and cause secondary damage beyond the original injury or infection. This is a particular problem with stroke or severe head injury, for example, and researchers are searching for ways to shut down this "inflammatory cascade."

By Invitation Only

One of the ways the immune system treats the brain differently is evident in the activity of B lymphocytes, the immune cells that patrol the body on the lookout for trouble and that mount an immediate attack if any is found. B cells do not freely enter the brain as they do most other organs but migrate there only after an immune response has been activated elsewhere in the body. It's as if the brain has locked its doorways to these immune cells, allowing them to enter only by special invitation, a process scientists do not yet fully understand. The blood-brain barrier, a fine mesh in the walls of the brain's blood vessels that prevents larger molecules in the blood from entering the brain, normally keeps immune cells, including B cells, at bay.

The brain even has its own exclusive army of sentinels, called microglia. These tiny cells can be thought of as highly trained specialists within the immune defense system, having evolved with the sole purpose of protecting the sensitive tissue of the brain without perturbing its complex nerve-cell connections and pathways. Microglia respond swiftly to an assault on the brain, sometimes migrating great distances to reach the battlefield, and wall off offending microbes or areas that have been damaged by disease or injury. Still, even microglia can spell trouble for delicate brain tissues, and scientists are trying to understand how their response to sites of injury or infection might itself cause damage to neural structures.

(Excerpted from *The Dana Sourcebook of Immunology: Resources for Secondary and Post-Secondary Teachers and Students,* Dan Gordon, editor. Dana Press, Washington, DC, 2005.)

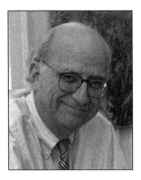

My Brain Made Me Do It

By Michael S. Gazzaniga, Ph.D.

As our ability to understand and change the brain increases, brain scientists and numerous other professionals are considering the effects on society that have arisen. A new field of study, neuroethics, has resulted. Here, Michael S. Gazzaniga, Ph.D., a leading neuroethicist, offers a very real scenario likely to confront someone serving as a juror. Dr. Gazzaniga extends beyond the courtroom questions that must be addressed by society as a whole.

Imagine being a juror on a horrific murder case. As a juror you know, or should know, some things about America's judicial system. First, 95 percent of criminal cases never come to trial; most cases are either dismissed or plea-bargained. The latter resolution is in part driven by the fact that courts tell defendants that, should they be found guilty at trial, the punishment will be more severe. Second, there is a huge probability the defendant is guilty.

When you take your seat in the jury box, you also know you'll have to decide the case with eleven of your peers, people who may not be up on the latest scientific understanding about

human behavior. You know most jurors don't buy excuses, facts presented about a defendant in an effort to claim he or she is exculpable for the crime at hand. Jurors are tough, practical people. That is the profile of the American jury system. Nothing fancy, just twelve people trying to make sense out of a horrible event. Most have never heard the word *neuroscience* or given a moment's thought to the concept of "free will." They are there to find out whether the defendant committed the crime, and if they determine he did, they will probably throw the book at him. Very few juries are asked to consider whether a defendant is exculpable for reasons of insanity, and when they do hear such a defense, they usually don't buy it.

Against this real backdrop of what life is like in the American courthouse, a new wrinkle is appearing in the form of the perennial question: Do we as a species have "free will"? Did the defendant carry out the horrible crime freely and by choice, or was it inevitable because of the nature of his brain and his past experiences? As with so many issues where modern scientific thinking confronts everyday realities, the people in the jury box are not rushing to embrace this one. Yet it is my contention that even those tough jurors will have no choice, because some day the issue will dominate the entire legal system.

Brain mechanisms are being explored that help us understand the role of genes in building our brains, the role of neuronal systems in allowing us to sense our environment, and the role of experience in guiding our future actions. We now understand that changes in our brain are both necessary and sufficient for changes in our mind. Indeed, an entire subfield of neuroscience, called cognitive neuroscience, has arisen in recent years to study the mechanisms of this occurrence.

With this reality of twenty-first-century brain science, many people find themselves worrying about those old chestnuts—free will and personal responsibility. The logic goes like this: The brain determines the mind, and the brain is a physical entity, subject to all the rules of the physical world. The physical world is determined, so our brains must also be determined. If our brains are determined, and the brain is the necessary and sufficient organ that enables the mind, we are then left with these questions: Are the thoughts that arise from our mind also determined? Is the free will we seem to experience just an illusion? And if free will is an illusion, must we revise our concepts of what it means to be personally responsible for our actions?

(Excerpted from *The Ethical Brain*, by Michael S. Gazzaniga. Dana Press, Washington, DC, 2005.)

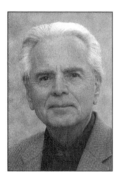

Out of the Blue

By Edward J. Sylvester

As a patient or visitor, most of us have watched medical specialists go about their life-saving work in a hospital. Science journalist Edward J. Sylvester has documented the work of a new type of medical professional, the neurointensivist, who works on cases of severe brain trauma or injury. In that setting, Sylvester details the roles of two more traditional brain doctors, the neurosurgeon and the neurologist, and their roles in saving the lives of brain-injured patients.

The neurosurgeon and neurologist are in many ways opposite personalities drawn together by a common obsession—an obsession with "neuro," the brain. Neurosurgeons study brain scans of every type available, picturing in their minds what these projections of the three-dimensional brain will look like close at hand, in light brighter than day. That is their defining moment: *there is the brain,* and they have to deal with it. Neurosurgery is a specialty only a century old. For half that time, in terrain where major structures are measured in millimeters and crucial vessels are the size of a hair, its morbidity and mortality rates were so high that truly elective neurosurgery was rare. The introduction of the intraoperative microscope in the 1960s began a revolution that empowered those with the skills and the patience and fortitude to use them. The only way to appreciate the difficulty of that job—other than spending seven years in residency learning it—is to watch it up close, often.

Neurosurgery requires an intensity of focus over many hours that is perhaps unmatched in medicine, where focus is always critical. Yet neurosurgeons live to operate. Rafael Tamargo, a top vascular neurosurgeon, had been dismayed for years by the number of elective patients who had to be turned away from Johns Hopkins to find other hospitals, for lack of [neuro intensive care unit] beds to support their neurosurgeries. "Last year we had 58 turnbacks," he said to [Marek A. Mirski, M.D., Ph.D., head of the Neuro ICU at Johns Hopkins Hospital in Baltimore] one day recently. The pain of those lost elective cases—lost rescues—was palpable for someone like Tamargo, ordinarily full of good humor and optimism. Neurosurgeons may run the gamut in terms of good humor or lack of it, but optimism is a defining trait. If healing could be willed by faith and positive thinking, neurosurgery would have no bad outcomes. With the expansion of the Neuro ICU, the neurosurgeons were hoping for no turnbacks. The terrain that vascular neurosurgeons dwell in is as complex as any known, even relative to other areas of neurosurgery....

But the neurosurgeon's ability to see, touch, and fix the brain as an object in space also illuminates just how hard the neurologists' job is. The neurologist's defining actions start today, as centuries ago, when a patient presents with symptoms that their experience tells them can be traced into the brain. The neurologist observes, ponders, hypothesizes—then studies all the most-modern scans as ardently as the surgeon, for confirmation or rejection, for nuance and detail—for conclusion, if possible. Nevertheless, you will hear many of the neurologists attending here in the intensive care unit remind fellows and residents that no scan can replace "the neurological exam." It is the neurologist's trademark, an entire program of examination of physical responses to questions, to touches, to probe movements so subtle in what they tell the experienced practitioner, that the neuro exam reveals deficits hours or days before they become visible on any scan. What is the point of predicting the future? To alter it.

Here, for now, is the ultimate scan: Read millions of bits of information coming out of this sealed dome and deduce from them what is going on inside. Then figure from that reading what will happen; take steps to prevent the bad and enhance the good—all without literally going in there.

(Excerpted from *Back from the Brink: How Crises Spur Doctors to New Discoveries about the Brain,* by Edward J. Sylvester. Dana Press, Washington, DC, 2004.)

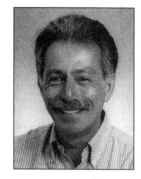
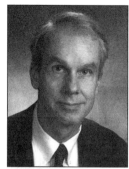
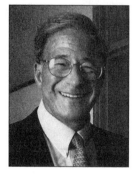

Behind the Scenes in the Adolescent Brain

Floyd E. Bloom, M.D., M. Flint Beal, M.D., and David J. Kupfer, M.D., Editors

Adolescence has been described as a busy time for the human brain. It's a time of transition as the brain, like the rest of the body, physically eases into adulthood and, in the process, the brain's gray matter absorbs an explosion of new external stimuli. In this article, the authors look at the unique external and internal developments of the teenage years: high school, peer pressure, sexuality. The list goes on, and as it does, the brain is challenged. In most cases it thrives; sometimes it does not.

A large part of adolescent development takes place in the *frontal lobes,* which house an incredible number of faculties that we use many times each day. Here are the brain sites that enable us to make sense of the floods of information constantly being gathered by our five senses; to know when we are experiencing an emotion, and even to think about it while we feel it; to understand and keep track of the passage of time; and to hold a thought or object briefly in the forefront of our mind while we proceed with another thought (an ability known as working memory). According to a recent animal study of frontal lobe development, several different "transporter" molecules, which help the neurons to take in neurotransmitter molecules and break them down for reuse, either increase in density during adolescence or reach a plateau, which in turn alters some signaling pathways and stabilizes others. Partly from refinements in the signal circuits of the frontal lobes and partly through accumulated experience, adolescence gradually brings greater independence along with new capacities to plan, to consider the possible consequences of an action, and to take responsibility for the conduct of one's life.

Not surprisingly for a major executive center, the frontal lobes must reorganize to meet new demands, and they do so at more than one level in the years leading up to adulthood. One of the most significant changes (which actually continues well into adulthood) is a major increase in the myelination, or insulation, of the nerve fibers going both into and out of the frontal lobes. Greater insulation here means faster signaling, and perhaps more highly branched signaling pathways, between frontal lobe neurons and those in any distant region of the brain. This is a development that we can understand on an everyday level. Clearly, the more information the executive center can gather in various modes—visual signals, the emphatic tone of someone's voice, the emotions of the moment—the more nuanced and appropriate the brain's responses can be.

At a day-to-day level, adolescents encounter increasing demands on their attention. For starters, entering middle school or high school means a lot more to keep track of. Instead of being with one teacher in one classroom all day, students move among a half-dozen different classrooms, with a homeroom somewhere else

and a locker at yet another place. And, typically today, it quickly becomes necessary to juggle various homework assignments and projects and to balance them against sports or after-school activities, paid or volunteer work, and an ever more complicated social life. Is it any wonder that researchers, psychologists, and sociologists alike are becoming concerned about the long-term effects of these very crowded schedules on the young, developing brain? Some experts warn that our society may be overencouraging the development of quick responses and mental multitasking in young people, at the expense of equally valuable life skills: planning, thinking things through, and predicting the consequences of actions.

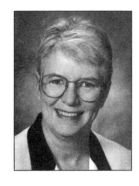 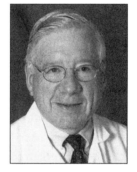

Defining Stroke or Brain Attack

By Cleo Hutton and Louis R. Caplan, M.D.

Stroke, or brain attack, is the third leading cause of death in the United States. Cleo Hutton's account of surviving a stroke is complemented by medical and scientific commentary from a leading expert in the field, Louis R. Caplan, M.D. Dr. Caplan explains Hutton's case in terms of what scientists and doctors have come to know about strokes.

The term stroke describes brain injury caused by an abnormality of the blood supply to a part of the brain. The word is derived from the fact that most sufferers are struck suddenly by the vascular abnormality. Abnormalities of brain function begin quickly, sometimes within an instant. *Stroke* is a very broad term that describes several different types of vascular diseases involving the blood vessels that supply the brain with needed nourishment and fuel. Since treatment depends on the type of stroke and the blood vessels involved, it is very important for the doctor to determine precisely what caused the vascular and brain injury and where the abnormalities are located.

Strokes fall into two very broad groups: ischemia and hemorrhage. Cleo had the most common type of stroke—ischemia—which means a lack of blood. Hemorrhage and ischemia are polar opposites: in hemorrhage, too much blood collects inside the skull; in ischemia, there is not enough blood supply to allow survival of the affected brain tissue. About four strokes out of every five are ischemic. When a part of the brain is not getting adequate blood, it may stop performing its usual tasks. A good comparison is the fuel pump in a car. If a fuel line is blocked and you step on the gas pedal, the car will not go because of the lack of fuel. But when the fuel line opens, the car will return to its normal behavior—and the car is not necessarily damaged. When the blood supply to a part of the brain is deficient for enough time, the tissue dies. The death of tissue caused by ischemia is called infarction. With *CT scans* we can tell whether the brain contains a hemorrhage, which looks white on the scan, or an infarct, which shows damage as black or gray....

There are three major categories of brain ischemia: thrombosis, embolism, and systemic hypoperfusion. Each indicates a different reason for decreased blood flow. I find these terms easiest to explain by comparing them with house plumbing. Suppose that one day you turn on the faucet in the bathroom on the second floor and no water comes out, or it comes out in an inadequate drip. The problem could be a local one, such as a rust buildup in the pipe leading to that sink. This is analogous to *thrombosis*, a term used to describe a local process occurring in one blood vessel region. Atherosclerosis or another disease narrows the artery. When the artery becomes very narrow, the resulting change in blood flow causes blood to clot, resulting in total occlusion of the artery. Clearly this is a local problem in one pipe; a plumber would attempt to fix the blocked pipe. Similarly, physicians treat a narrowed (stenosed) or occluded artery by trying to open it or by creating a detour around it.

But a blocked pipe to a second-floor sink could also be caused by debris in the water system that came to rest in that pipe, rather than by a local problem that began within the pipe. When particles break loose and block a distant artery, we call it an embolism. (The place where the material originates is called the donor site; the receiving artery is the recipient site; and the material is called an embolus.) An artery within the head can be blocked by a blood clot or other particles that break loose from the heart, from the aorta (the major artery leading away from the heart), or from one of the major arteries in the neck or head. An embolism was the cause of Cleo's stroke.

Suppose instead that the plumber finds that the water did not flow normally in your second floor sink because the water pressure in your house is intermittently low and flow to all sinks and showers is faulty due to a leak in the water tank or low water pressure in the entire house plumbing. This situation is like systemic hypoperfusion: there is no local problem within the pipe to one sink, but instead a general circulatory problem. Ischemia can be caused by inadequate pumping of blood from the heart or a low volume of blood or fluid in the body.

(Excerpted from *Striking Back at Stroke: A Doctor-Patient Journal*, by Cleo Hutton and Louis R. Caplan, M.D. Dana Press, Washington, DC, 2003.)

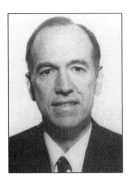

What Exactly Are Antidepressants?

By J. Raymond DePaulo, Jr., M.D.

Depression, in its unipolar form, may be the leading cause of disability worldwide; in its bipolar form—often called manic-depressive illness—it has both stimulated the creativity and diminished the will to live of some of the world's most brilliant artists, poets, scientists, and statesmen. J. Raymond DePaulo, Jr., M.D., professor of psychiatry at Johns Hopkins University School of Medicine, an active clinician, teacher, and researcher, has described depression as "a mystery disease," a paradoxical characterization of an illness for which brain science has produced an array of usually effective medications.

For all their differences, the many types of medications we call antidepressants are consistently better than placebo tablets in reducing symptoms in depressed patients. These medications do not, however, have the capacity to change anyone's personality, but rather act to restore the normal chemistry in the brain. Antidepressants go by many names based on their chemical structure or activity, such as the tricyclic structure or the *serotonin reuptake* inhibitor activity; that's not to suggest that every drug with a tricyclic structure and every drug that affects serotonin reuptake is necessarily an antidepressant. While demonstrating antidepressant activity, almost all these medications have other useful properties, particularly in anxiety disorders or in the regulation of blood pressure. That's why the word antidepressant can be confusing. I prefer to describe these medications in terms of their structure or function; for example, this drug affects serotonin or norepinephrine in this or that way.

The drugs we call antidepressants fall into four basic categories: tricyclics, selective serotonin reuptake inhibitors (SSRIs), monoamine oxidase inhibitors (MAOIs), and a number of newer drugs we can lump together under the necessarily vague designation of "others."

Serendipity has played an interesting role in the development of drugs that are currently being used to treat depressive illness. Swiss researchers were trying to make a better antihistamine when they created a compound containing a property that proved very helpful in treating psychotics and schizophrenics. The drug they created turned out to be Thorazine. Then, when researchers sought to make a better Thorazine they produced not an antipsychotic (a drug used to treat severe mental illness), but a tricyclic drug called imipramine. While imipramine didn't help people suffering from manias or schizophrenia, it did help people with depression. Once the tricyclics began to enjoy wide acceptance, pharmacists went back into the labs to attempt to make a better imipramine; they instead came up with Tegretol (also called carbamazepine), the first anticonvulsant mood stabilizer not derived from lithium. But happy accidents, as we all know, rarely happen in a vacuum. The discoverers of these compounds were astute enough to know how to see things they weren't looking for directly, and that's hard to do....

While there are differences between types of antidepressants, they are outweighed by their similarities. In fact, some experts have argued that, when you come right down to it, all antidepressants are basically the same, not only because the response rates are so similar, but because the chemical structure of these various drugs is much the same and the drugs overlap in terms of activity. Generally speaking, these drugs act by blocking the reuptake of neurotransmitters such as serotonin and norepinephrine in varying degrees.

These drugs leave more of the signal-carrying neurotransmitter "out there" in the brain rather than allowing so much of it to be sucked back into the neurons and produce mental or emotional problems. Keep in mind that altering chemical balances in the brain is what these drugs do, and while they often evoke a favorable response in that the patient feels much better over time, what makes these drugs work, what their exact mechanism is in the brain that has an effect on depression, remains a mystery.

(Excerpted from *Understanding Depression: What We Know and What You Can Do About It,* by J. Raymond DePaulo, Jr., M.D., with Leslie Alan Horvitz. Dana Press and John Wiley & Sons, Inc., New York, 2002.)

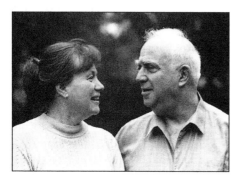

The Developing Nervous System: Vision

By Norbert Herschkowitz, M.D., and Elinore Chapman Herschkowitz

Norbert Herschkowitz, M.D., and his educator-writer wife, Elinore Chapman Herschkowitz, study how brain development shapes a child's personality, beginning with conception. Here they discuss visual development, a feat of information processing whose complexity we are still learning to appreciate. Scientists now know that some circuits of the visual system are up and running even before we are born.

The view really isn't much, perhaps at most a faint orange glow during the last weeks before birth. But even in the dark, your baby's visual system is under intense construc-

tion to prepare her for her life in the world of light. Already at around one month after fertilization, when the first traces of her brain as a whole come into view, tiny bulges that will become the baby's eyes appear.

Carla J. Shatz, now chair of the Department of Neurobiology at Harvard Medical School, showed in animal experiments that the basic wiring of the visual system begins to take place before any stimulation from the outside world reaches the baby's eyes. In the absence of light, special nerve cells in the retina of the eye called ganglion cells begin, probably under genetic influences, to fire off short bursts of electrical impulses. The impulses are transmitted from the retina along the optic nerve to the brain. The spontaneous electrical activity of these retina cells seems to be crucial for setting up the correct wiring. If it does not take place, vision will not develop normally.

The impressive groundwork takes place all by itself without any extra outside stimulation. However, adverse environmental conditions may prevent necessary developmental steps from taking place. The spontaneous firing of the nerve cells in the visual system is vulnerable to disruptions. Drugs that interfere with the transmission of electrical activity across the synapse (e.g., nicotine, benzodiazepines, or narcotics) could disturb the pattern of the fine connections and lead to later visual deficits.

By the time your baby is born, her visual system is basically set up. But it will need the stimulation of the outside world to complete the job—and there is plenty out there waiting....

Looking Around

Once your baby has taken his first breath or two, his eyes blink at all the bright light in the delivery room and he stares astounded by all the unfamiliar sights. Now his sense of vision suddenly becomes important for helping him become acquainted with his world. While his sense of hearing has been exposed to a great variety of sounds in the uterus and his sense of touch has been stimulated by contacts with his own body or the uterine wall, his visual system has been pretty much left in the dark until now.

Newborn babies seem eager to find out what's going on. Marshall Haith and his colleagues observed infants lying in a dark room. Even in complete darkness, the infants' eyes moved around as if they were looking for something to attract their attention. Since no light was entering the babies' eyes, the investigators concluded that the eye movements were "endogenous," that is, the result of direct activity of the brain rather than of outside stimulation.

A newborn baby sees faces as blurred figures surrounded by areas of light, and the baby's eyes can focus only on objects that are within about 8 to 30 inches. That is about the distance between a mother's face and that of her baby when she is holding him during feeding.

Newborns focus on strong lines and distinct contours. Studies have shown that they can tell the difference between the outline shapes of a triangle, square, circle, and cross. In human faces, the eyes and hairline are prominent features. Perhaps for this reason, mothers—and fathers—of newborn infants might think twice about changing their hairstyles too often.

(Excerpted from *A Good Start in Life: Understanding Your Child's Brain and Behavior from Birth to Age 6,* by Norbert Herschkowitz, M.D., and Elinore Chapman Herschkowitz. Dana Press/Joseph Henry Press, Washington, DC, 2002.)

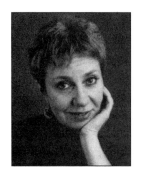

The Science of Attracting Axons—The Final Key to Spinal Cord Regeneration?

By Luba Vikhanski

For millennia, scientists and doctors have viewed damage to the spinal cord as permanent. Science journalist Luba Vikhanski writes that startling new discoveries in the last 20 years have greatly improved our understanding of the "wiring" process of the fetal nervous system and opened a window on the workings of the mature spinal cord. Treatment and cures from this and other research paths could follow.

As befits a mechanism perfected over 600 million years, axonal guidance is a smoothly scripted affair. *Axons* travel a long distance, sometimes more than a thousand times greater than the diameter of their cell bodies, before settling into their assigned spots. They negotiate this challenging journey by breaking it up into short segments, each perhaps a fraction of a millimeter long. At the end of each segment, the growth cone appears to pause, like a traveler at a crossroads, making navigating decisions. What helps it choose its course is the presence of guidance chemicals.…

Axons have no problem following the attractive and repulsive cues in the embryo, but by adulthood something happens to the environment in the central nervous system, making it hostile to growth. Scientists hypothesize that the "go" signs that guided axons to the places in the fetus turn into "stop" signs in the adult organism. To produce regeneration, the guiding signs would have to be switched from "stop" back to "go." This idea is based on a fascinating property of all guidance molecules: They can be attractive or repellent at different times, or attractive for some growth cones but repulsive for others, which suggests that their guiding properties can be manipulated.

Scientists have proposed that the molecular "stop-go" switch may be the same for all guidance molecules. No one has yet proved this hypothesis, but in several studies a manipulation of guiding properties has already been accomplished. In one series of experiments, a team led by Dr. Mu-ming Poo, from the University of California at San Diego, in collaboration with [Dr. Marc] Tessier-Lavigne's lab, achieved a feat that sounds like an episode from a romantic novel. The scientists managed to transform repulsion into attraction. Using a molecular switch they identified, they altered the effect of two guidance molecules on the tips of growing nerve fibers: Instead of repelling the growing fibers, the molecules started to attract the fibers in a laboratory dish.

Scientists are trying to identify the key targets for such manipulation. Netrins, first identified in worms and chick embryos but later found to be present in fruit flies and in humans, are among the potential candidates. Timothy Kennedy, former postdoctoral fellow from Tessier-Lavigne's San Francisco netrin team, who now runs his own lab at McGill University's Montreal Neurological Institute, has shown with his colleagues that netrins are present in large amounts in the adult spinal cord of rats, and that their amounts change after injury. During development, netrins have been shown to attract the growth of some axons and repel the growth of others, but Kennedy believes that their role in the adult nervous system may be to block nerve fiber growth. By cranking up the attractive properties of netrins, he suggests, it may be possible to encourage spinal cord axons to regenerate in adults.

(Excerpted from *In Search of the Lost Cord: Solving the Mystery of Spinal Cord Regeneration,* by Luba Vikhanski. Dana Press/Joseph Henry Press, Washington, DC, 2001.)

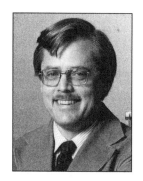

Allostatic Load Scenario 4: Too Little Is as Bad as Too Much

By Bruce S. McEwen, Ph.D.

Stress is just one of among a host of factors that contribute to what we call "allostatic load," says Bruce McEwen, Ph.D., professor of neuroendocrinology at the Rockefeller University. Dr. McEwen defines allostasis as "the ability of the body to achieve stability through its own regulatory changes." Allostasis is affected by diet, sleep, exercise, whether or not we drink or smoke, and even our socioeconomic status. "If our allostatic load is high, our bodies work overtime to maintain balance."

The idea of checks and balances in the stress response brings us to the final way in which the protective systems of allostatis can trigger the damage of allostatic load: when the stress response is insufficient, resulting in underproduction of the stress hormones, particularly *cortisol*, wear and tear can also result....How can this be? Surely if there are no stress hormones, there must be no stress and consequently no stress-related illness. But like most of human physiology, it isn't quite that simple. Cortisol acts somewhat like a thermostat; in fact, it clamps down on its own production. It slows the production of the two hormones that touch off the HPA (*hypothalamus-pituitary-adrenal*) axis: corticotropin-releasing factor in the hypothalamus and adreno-corticotropic hormone in the pituitary. Cortisol also reins in the immune system and reduces inflammation and swelling from tissue damage.

When one of the participants in a checks-and-balances arrangement isn't doing its job, the others may go overboard in doing theirs. In some people, allostatic load takes the form of a sluggish response by the adrenals and a subsequent lack of sufficient cortisol. The most immediate result is that the immune system, without cortisol's steadying hand, runs wild and reacts to things that do not really pose a threat to the body. Allergies are one example of this process. In most people the immune system does not put things like dust and cat dander on a par with pathogenic (disease-causing) bacteria. But in people prone to allergies, the immune system goes on red alert in the presence of such usually innocuous sub-stances, throwing everything it's got at the irri-tants: uncontrollable sneezing to expel the invaders, mucous secretion to entrap them, swelling caused by the influx of white blood cells to the infected area, pain, redness, and general misery. All of these symptoms are reduced by the action of cortisol....

A feeble HPA response can often manifest itself in conditions not always immediately asso-ciated with the immune system. Fibromyalgia, for example, is a condition of chronic pain that most doctors consider psychosomatic (and some con-sider imaginary, though the patients certainly don't). The connection with the immune system and cortisol becomes clear when we consider that pain is a part of the inflammatory response; pain warns us that there's a problem and encourages us to leave the affected area alone until the prob-lem is resolved. But in many chronic pain states, as with other inflammatory disorders, there is no apparent threat. Rather, the system is responding in a maladaptive way, which the available supply of cortisol is too low to prevent.

(Excerpted from *The End of Stress as We Know It*, by Bruce McEwen, with Elizabeth N. Lasley. Dana Press/Joseph Henry Press, Washington, DC, 2002.)

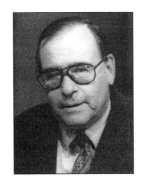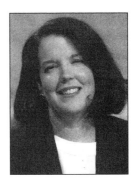

Research and Future Treatments for Alzheimer's Disease

By Guy S. McKhann, M.D., and Marilyn Albert, Ph.D.

Alzheimer's disease expert Dennis J. Selkoe, M.D., has written, "In the past few years, we have not only identified the genes that cause Alzheimer's, we are also beginning to understand how they work. In their mutated forms, every one of the Alzheimer's genes that scientists have discovered work by subtly different mechanisms to increase the amount of amyloid beta-protein in the brain." Two of the world's leading neu-rological experts, Marilyn Albert, Ph.D., formerly of Harvard University and Guy McKhann, M.D., of Johns Hopkins University, take a detailed look at the promising outlook for treating one of our most notori-ous medical disorders.

It is imperative that ways to prevent and treat this disease be found. If prevention efforts could delay the average onset of the disease by only five years, it would have enormous impact. If the sharp increase in numbers of cases could be delayed until people reached age 90, many peo-ple would die of other causes before they ever got Alzheimer's disease.

Every pharmaceutical company worth its salt is therefore working on how to slow the progres-sion or delay the first symptoms of Alzheimer's disease. In general they are working in several basic areas. The first approach is to prevent the accumulation of the abnormal form of amyloid protein. These fragments, called AB or A-beta, vary in length, but one particular length is especially toxic to nerve cells. Researchers are concentrating on either preventing this toxic fragment from accumulating or removing it from the brain. Genetically engineered "Alzheimer mice," who show the same toxic buildup in their brains as human patients do, are invaluable to this research....

The second approach involves getting the body to use its immune system to remove the amyloid from the brain. A person is injected, that is immunized, with the offending fragment of amyloid, and then makes antibodies to this fragment. The person's own antibodies attack and remove the amyloid. In the Alzheimer mice, the antibodies not only removed the amyloid plaques, they kept them from forming.

A third approach is to try to keep alive the nerve cells in which amyloid is already accumulating. Two agents are currently being studied: vitamin E and estrogen. Substances called trophic factors also may help sustain these endangered cells. The brain normally deploys trophic factors in very small quantities to maintain the health of nerve cells. With the techniques of *molecular biology*, researchers can now make large amounts of these substances and try them out as drugs for treatment. The problem is getting trophic factors into the areas of the brain affected by the disease. One approach is to use genetic engineering—to put the gene that directs the production of the trophic factor into a bacterium that's been rendered harmless, then put the bacterium into the brain to deliver the gene to the brain cells. This sounds like science fiction but actually works in experimental animals. Preliminary trials of this gene therapy are under way in people.

The final strategy is to decrease the inflammation in the brain that occurs in response to the abnormal amyloid's attack on nerve cells. This approach takes its cue from recent advances in treating arthritis' inflammation in the joints with anti-inflammatory medications like aspirin, Motrin, or the recently FDA-approved COX-2

inhibitors. Studies are ongoing to see if these anti-inflammatory drugs have a role in treating Alzheimer's disease.

(Excerpted from *Keep Your Brain Young: The Complete Guide to Physical and Emotional Health and Longevity,* by Guy M. McKhann, M.D., and Marilyn S. Albert, Ph.D. Dana Press and John Wiley & Sons, Inc., New York, 2002.)

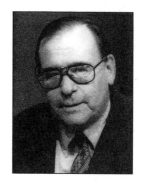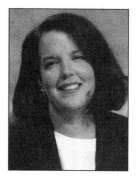

How Your Brain Forms Memories

By Guy S. McKhann, M.D., and Marilyn Albert, Ph.D.

How can physical matter, atoms and molecules, amassed in however intricate an arrangement in the three pounds of tissue that make up the human brain, retain for short periods, or for decades, the color and taste and smell of a ripe apple or the thought that the universe is curved? For centuries, this query has remained one of the most profound questions for science. The first Nobel Prize in Physiology or Medicine of the 21st century went to three neuroscientists, Eric R. Kandel, M.D.; Paul Greengard, Ph.D.; and Arvid Carlsson, M.D., in part for their fundamental work on memory formation. Drs. McKhann and Albert provide a closer look at memory here.

Can you drive your brain to be better than it is genetically programmed to be? Little evidence supports the possibility. However, it is clear that you can attain optimal functioning and maintain it by stimulating usage. Each nerve cell communicates with thousands of others. But when you form new memories, you strengthen a particular series of connections, the way a heavily trodden pathway in the woods becomes more visible and easier to follow. Among nerve cells, two different things are happening. First, changes take place in the physical connections between nerve cells to make one pathway easier to use than others. These changes occur at the very end of the pathway, at the synapses, where nerve cells connect with one another. Second, some of the chemicals released at the synapses, the neurotransmitters, are specialized for memory. One of these neurotransmitters is acetylcholine. Many of the drugs being developed to attempt to modify memory involve increasing the effectiveness of this neurotransmitter.

Mentally and physically stimulating activities promote this constant "rewiring" of the brain, strengthening its pathways and stimulating the production of substances required for the growth and maintenance of nerve cells. In some instances, brain cells will make new connections. More commonly the balance between existing connections is altered, by strengthening some and weakening others.

Years ago scientists thought of the brain as being "hard-wired," meaning that during development, nerve cells would assume their proper positions and make myriad interconnections. Once in place and interconnected, it was thought that nerve cells did not change. This notion is clearly wrong. Research in the last few years has shown that new nerve cells may even develop in areas of the adult brain, including the hippocampus, the area that is important for making new memories. No one knows what regulates this replenishment of nerve cells, but recent evidence suggests that one factor may be physical and mental activity.

Genetics of Memory

Genetics also plays a role in how well memory functions. The behavior of animals is a good example. Certain breeds of dog, such as Labradors, are supposed to be gentle but perhaps a little dumb, meaning they do not learn new information easily. German Shepherds, on the other hand, generally learn quickly but are not particularly gentle. The same phenomenon is well known in laboratory animals. Some strains of mice can be taught to find food in a maze much more easily than others. Now that we know that genes can be either more or less active, it is possible to breed mice that are selectively smart or dumb. This line of research is one of the approaches that may eventually lead to drugs that will enhance memory for people.

But what about us humans?…Some people may simply not have genetic vulnerabilities that lead to diseases like Alzheimer's disease. On the other hand, they may have other genes working that protect their brains from the decline in the ability of nerve cells to function normally. Research to explore these alternatives is already under way in animals, such as mice, in which the genetic properties can be manipulated.

(Excerpted from *Keep Your Brain Young: The Complete Guide to Physical and Emotional Health and Longevity,* by Guy M. McKhann, M.D., and Marilyn S. Albert, Ph.D. Dana Press and John Wiley & Sons, Inc., New York, 2002.)

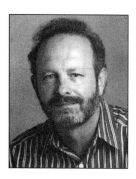

The Power of Emotions

By Joseph E. LeDoux, Ph.D.

New York University neuroscientist Joseph LeDoux, Ph.D., and other neuroscientists have begun to examine the way the brain shapes our experience—and our memories—to generate the varied repertoire of human emotions. Specifically, as Dr. LeDoux explains, he chose to begin his inquiry by examining an emotion that is common to all living creatures: fear.

Years of research by many workers have given us extensive knowledge of the neural pathways involved in processing acoustic information, which is an excellent starting point for examining the neurological foundations of fear. The natural flow of auditory information—the way you hear music, speech, or anything else—is that the sound comes into the ear, enters the brain, goes up to a region called the auditory midbrain, then to the auditory thalamus, and ultimately to the auditory cortex. Thus, in the auditory pathway, as in other sensory systems, the cortex is the highest level of processing.

So the first question we asked when we began these studies of the fear system was: Does the sound have to go all the way to the auditory cortex in order for the rat to learn that the sound paired with the shock is dangerous? When we made *lesions* in the auditory cortex, we found that the animal could still make the association between the sound and the shock, and would still react with fear behavior to the sound alone. Since information from all our senses is processed in the cortex—which ultimately allows us to become conscious of seeing the predator or hearing the sound—the fact that the cortex didn't seem to be necessary to fear conditioning was both intriguing and mystifying. We wanted to understand how something as important as the emotion of fear could be mediated by the brain if it wasn't going into the cortex, where all the higher processes occur. So we next made lesions in the auditory thalamus and then in the auditory midbrain. The midbrain supplies the major sensory input to the thalamus, which in turn supplies the major sensory input to the cortex. What we found was that lesions in either of these subcortical areas completely eliminated the rat's susceptibility to fear conditioning. If the lesions were made in an unconditioned rat, the animal could not learn to make the association between sound and shock, and if the lesions were made on a rat that had already been conditioned to fear the sound, it would no longer react to the sound.

But if the stimulus didn't have to reach the cortex, where was it going from the thalamus? Some other area or areas of the brain must receive information from the thalamus and establish memories about experiences that stimulate a fear response. To find out, we made a tracer injection in the auditory thalamus (the part of the thalamus that processes sounds) and found that some cells in this structure projected axons into the amygdala. This is key, because the amygdala has for many years been known to be important in emotional responses. So it appeared that information went to the amygdala from the thalamus without going to the neocortex.

We then did experiments with rats that had amygdala lesions, measuring freezing and blood-pressure responses elicited by the sound after conditioning. We found that the amygdala lesion prevented conditioning from taking place. In fact, the responses are very similar to those of unconditioned animals that hear the sound for the first time, without getting the shock.

So the amygdala is critical to this pathway.

It receives information about the outside world directly from the thalamus, and immediately sets in motion a variety of bodily responses. We call this thalamo-amygdala pathway the low road because it's not taking advantage of all of the higher-level information processing that occurs in the neocortex, which also communicates with the amygdala.

(Excerpted from *States of Mind: New Discoveries about How Our Brains Make Us Who We Are,* Roberta Conlan, editor. Dana Press and John Wiley & Sons, Inc., New York, 1999.)

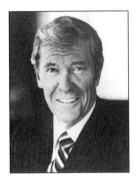 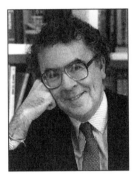

Use It or Lose It
Take Active Measures Now to Combat Disuse Atrophy

By David Mahoney and Richard M. Restak, M.D.

David Mahoney, businessman and philanthropist, and neurologist Richard Restak, M.D., point out that the 20th century's increase in life span (30 years longer average life expectancy) and spectacular gains in neuroscience and medicine will make the 100-year life span commonplace in another generation or two. This advance will happen only if we take proactive measures in such matters as handling stress properly and seeking out lifelong mental activity.

Certain cells in areas of the brain beneath the cortex (called subcortical nuclei) are sometimes irreverently dubbed the "juice machines." They give us enthusiasm and general "get up and go" energy. When Samuel Johnson said, "The question is not so much 'Is it worth seeing?' but rather 'Is it worth going to see?'" he was unknowingly referring to the subcortical nuclei, which generate enthusiasm and energy.

With aging, almost everyone undergoes some loss of cells in the subcortical nuclei. It's what we notice when we joke that our get-up-and-go "got up and went." Since this is natural, our task is to recognize that we are "mellowing" rather than losing any of our abilities. Our attention to those abilities, as intact as ever, helps us maintain mental vigor.

Every talent and special skill that you've developed over your lifetime is represented in your brain by a complex network of neurons. And each time you engage in any activity that involves your talents and skills, the neuronal linkages in that network are enhanced. Think of the brain cells as shaped like trees composed of long branches subdividing into smaller and smaller branches. As the result of brain growth and the person's experience in the world, tremendous overlap and connectivity develop among the tree branches. Neuroscientists, struck with the tree analogy, refer to this process as "arborization."

Eventually nerve cells form active circuits based on these branchlike linkages. The more often the circuits are activated, the easier it is to activate them the next time. Subjectively, you experience this as the formation of a habit. With time the activity gets easier to do; the more the skill or talent is practiced, the better you get at it. But if you neglect your talents and skills, they begin to wane, and over time it becomes harder and harder to perform at your best. If enough time passes you will experience great difficulty returning to your former level of excellence. That's because the neuronal circuits have fallen into disuse: greater degrees of effort are required to activate them. But no matter how long you've neglected a skill, you'll never find yourself in the same situation as the person who never learned the skill in the first place.

Neuronal circuits, once established, never

entirely disappear. It's the ease of facilitating them that varies. This law of facilitation and disuse atrophy applies to every activity, whether physical or mental. Neglect your tennis or your golf for enough time and your skills in these very different activities will deteriorate.

Remember that the brain is an ever-changing organ. If one part gets rusty and suffers atrophy from disuse, its functions are taken over by other areas that are used more. When we stop challenging ourselves and expanding, or at least maintaining our skills, the brain cells involved in the neuronal networks drop out and link into other networks. Eventually the skill has almost entirely disappeared. We say almost because some neurons, though a much smaller number, always remain in the network.

(Excerpted from *The Longevity Strategy: How to Live to 100 Using the Brain-Body Connection,* by David Mahoney and Richard Restak, M.D. Dana Press and John Wiley & Sons, Inc., New York, 1998. Mr. Mahoney died in 2000 at the age of 76.)

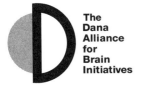 **The Dana Alliance for Brain Initiatives**

The Dana Alliance for Brain Initiatives represents a group of leading neuroscientists who commit themselves to translating advances in brain research to the public, the ultimate beneficiary of these advances. Dana Alliance members number more than 200, including ten Nobel laureates. They represent virtually every subspeciality within neuroscience. Their vision and goals statement, reprinted here in its entirety, outlines the potential for new treatments and therapies and speaks to the importance of continued basic research and the need to keep the public informed of progress in neuroscience.

Imagine a World

■ In which Alzheimer's, Parkinson's, and Lou Gehrig's (ALS) diseases and retinitis pigmentosa and other causes of blindness are commonly detected in their early stages, and are swiftly treated by medications that stop deterioration before significant damage occurs.

■ In which spinal cord injury doesn't mean a lifetime of paralysis because the nervous system can be programmed to rewire neural circuits and re-establish muscle movement.

■ In which drug addiction and alcoholism no longer hold people's lives hostage because easily available treatments can interrupt the changes in neural pathways that cause withdrawal from, and drive the craving for, addictive substances.

■ In which the genetic pathways and environmental triggers that predispose people to mental illness are understood so that accurate diagnostic tests and targeted therapies—including medications, counseling, and preventive interventions—are widely available and fully employed.

■ In which new knowledge about brain development is used to enhance the benefits of the crucial early learning years and combat diseases associated with aging.

■ In which people's daily lives are not compromised by attacks of depression or anxiety because better medications are developed to treat these conditions.

Although such a vision may seem unrealistic and utopian, we are at an extraordinarily exciting time in the history of neuroscience. The advances in research during the past decade have taken us further than we had imagined. We have expanded our understanding of the basic mechanisms of how the brain works, and are at a point where we can harness the healing potential of that knowledge.

We have already begun to devise strategies, new technologies, and treatments to combat a range of neurological diseases and disorders. By setting therapeutic goals, and applying what we know, we will develop effective treatments—and, in some instances, cures.

For all that has been learned in neuroscience recently, we are learning how much we do not know. That creates the urgency to continue basic research that looks at the broader questions of how living things work. This will help to formulate the complex questions that lead to scientific discovery.

Public confidence in science is essential if we are to be successful in our mission. To this end we recognize that dialogue between researchers and the public will be essential in considering the ethical and social consequences of advances in brain research.

The Dana Alliance for Brain Initiatives and the European Dana Alliance for the Brain represent a community of neuroscientists willing to commit to ambitious goals, as seen in 1992 in Cold Spring Harbor, New York, where an American research agenda was set forth, and again in 1997 when the newly formed European group followed suit with its own goals and objectives. Both groups now are moving to build upon gains made so far. We are setting new goals to guide what can be achieved in the near term, and to project even further into the future. By allowing ourselves to imagine what benefit to humanity this new era in neuroscience is likely to bring, we can speed progress toward achieving our goals.

The coordinated work of thousands of basic and clinical scientists in multiple disciplines, ranging from molecular structure and drug design to genomics, brain imaging, cognitive science, and clinical investigation, has given us a pool of information that we can now build into therapeutic applications for all neurological diseases and disorders. As scientists, we will continue to move forward not just as individuals, exploring our particular areas of interest, but also in concert with colleagues in all areas of science, mining opportunities to collaborate across disciplines.

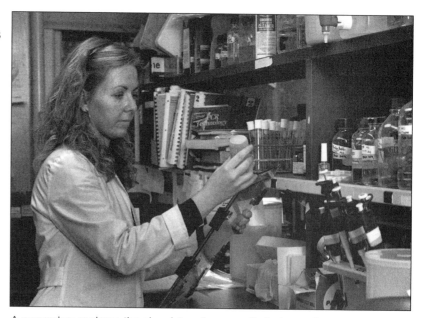

A researcher analyzes the chemistry of nerve cells that coordinate with muscles to produce movement.

Our Commitment, Bench to Bedside

Today, neuroscience research benefits from an unprecedented breadth of opportunity. We have expanded our understanding of brain function, disease onset, and disease progression. A sophisticated arsenal of tools and techniques now enables us to apply our knowledge and to accelerate progress in brain research.

As scientists, we are committed to continue making progress "at the bench." To attack major brain disorders such as Alzheimer's, stroke, or Parkinson's will require continued basic research from which clinicians can move toward development of new treatments and therapies. We have a responsibility to continue such research and to enlist its support by the public.

We also have the obligation to explain those areas of scientific research that soon may have direct application to human beings. To progress beyond laboratory research, we need to take the next clinical steps in partnership with the public—translating science into real and genuine benefits "at the bedside."

As our tools and techniques become more sophisticated, they may be considered threatening in their perceived potential for misuse. It is important to recognize the understandable fears that brain research may allow scientists to alter the most important aspects of our brains and behavior, changing the very things that make us uniquely human. Public confidence in the integrity of scientists, in the safety of clinical trials—the cornerstone of applied research—and in the assurance of patient confidentiality must be continually maintained.

Putting research into a real-life context is always a challenge. People not only want to know how and why research is done, they also want to know why it matters to them. Allaying the public's concerns that the findings of brain science could be used in ways that might be harmful or ethically questionable is particularly important. Meeting both of these challenges is essential if those affected by neurological or psychiatric disorders are to reap fully the benefits of brain research.

Our mission as neuroscientists has to go beyond brain research. We accept our responsibility to explain in plain language where our science and its new tools and techniques are likely to take us. We, the members of the Dana Alliance and the European Dana Alliance, willingly embrace this mission as we embark on a new decade of hope, hard work, and partnership with the public.

The Goals

Combat the devastating impact of Alzheimer's disease.

In Alzheimer's disease, a small piece of the amyloid protein accumulates and is toxic to nerve cells. The mechanism of this accumulation has been worked out biochemically and in genetic studies in animals. Using these *animal models,* new therapeutic drugs and a potentially powerful vaccine are being developed to prevent the accumulation of this toxic material or enhance its removal. These new therapies, which will be tried in humans in the near future, offer realistic hope that this disease process can be effectively treated.

Discover how best to treat Parkinson's disease.

Drugs that act on *dopamine* pathways in the brain have had significant success in treating the motor abnormalities of Parkinson's disease. Unfortunately, this therapeutic benefit wears off for many patients after 5 to 10 years. New drugs are being developed to prolong the action of dopamine-based treatments and to slow the selective loss of nerve cells that causes this disease. For those in whom drug therapies fail, surgical approaches, such as deep brain stimulation, are likely to be of benefit. Newer forms of brain imaging have made it possible to determine if these treatments are rescuing nerve cells and restoring their circuits back toward normal.

Decrease the incidence of stroke and improve post-stroke therapies.

Heart disease and stroke can be strikingly reduced when people stop smoking, keep their cholesterol levels low, and maintain normal weight by diet and exercise, and when diabetes is detected and treated. For those with strokes, rapid evaluation and treatment can lead to dramatic improvement and less disability. New treatments will be developed to further reduce the acute impact of stroke on normal brain cells. New rehabilitation techniques, based on understanding how the brain adjusts itself following injury, will result in further improvement.

Develop more successful treatments for mood disorders such as depression, schizophrenia, obsessive-compulsive disorder, and bipolar disorder.

Although the genes for these diseases have eluded researchers over the past decade, the sequencing of the human genome will reveal several of the genes for these conditions. New imaging techniques, along with new knowledge about the actions of these genes in the brain, will make it possible to see how certain brain circuits go awry in these disorders of mood and thought. This will provide the basis for better diagnosis of patients, more effective use of today's medications, and the development of entirely new agents for treatment.

Uncover genetic and neurobiological causes of epilepsy and advance its treatment.

Understanding the genetic roots of epilepsy and the neural mechanisms that cause seizures will provide opportunities for preventive diagnosis and targeted therapies. Advances in electronic and surgical therapies promise to provide valuable treatment options.

Discover new and effective ways to prevent and treat multiple sclerosis.

For the first time, we have drugs that can modify the course of this disease. New drugs, aimed at altering the body's immune responses, will continue to decrease the number and severity of attacks of multiple sclerosis. New approaches will be taken to stop the longer-term progression caused by the breakdown of nerve fibers.

Develop better treatments for brain tumors.

Many types of brain tumors, especially those that are malignant or have spread from cancer outside the brain, are difficult to treat. Imaging techniques, focused-radiation treatments, different forms of delivery of drugs to the tumor, and the identification of genetic markers that will assist diagnosis should provide the basis for development of innovative therapies.

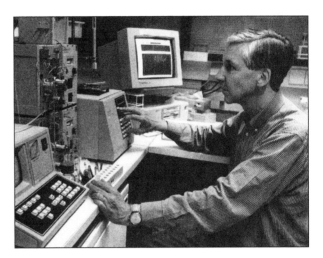

Improve recovery from traumatic brain and spinal cord injuries.

Treatments are being evaluated that decrease the amount of injured tissue immediately after an injury. Other agents are aimed at promoting the rewiring of nerve fibers. Techniques that encourage cellular regeneration in the brain to replace dead and damaged neurons will advance from animal models to human clinical trials. Electronic prostheses are being developed that use microchip technology to control neural circuits and return movement to paralyzed limbs.

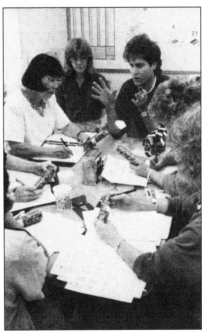

Create new approaches for pain management.

Pain, as a medical condition, need no longer be woefully undertreated. Research into the causation of pain and the neural mechanisms that drive it will give neuroscientists the tools they need to develop more effective and more highly targeted therapies for pain relief.

Treatments and cures for some of our most devastating, chronic disorders will be found in brain research and public support for it.

Treat addiction at its origins in the brain.

Researchers have identified the neural circuits involved in every known drug of abuse, and have cloned major receptors for these drugs. Advances in brain imaging, by identifying the neurobiological mechanisms that turn a normal brain into an addicted brain, will enable us to develop therapies that can either reverse or compensate for these changes.

Understand the brain mechanisms underlying the response to stress, anxiety, and depression.

Good mental health is a prerequisite for a good quality of life. Stress, anxiety, and depression not only damage people's lives, they can also have a devastating impact on society. As we come to understand the body's response to stress and the brain circuits implicated in anxiety and depression, we will be able to develop more effective ways to prevent them, and better treatments to lessen their impact.

The Strategy

Take advantage of the findings of genomic research.

The complete sequence of all the genes that comprise the human genome will soon be available. This means that we will be able, within the next 10 to 15 years, to determine which genes are active in each region of the brain under different functional states, and at every stage in life—from early embryonic life, through infancy, adoles-

cence, and throughout adulthood. It will be possible to identify which genes are altered so that their protein products are either missing or functioning abnormally in a variety of neurological and psychiatric disorders. Already this approach has enabled scientists to establish the genetic basis of such disorders as Huntington's disease, the spinocerebellar ataxias, muscular dystrophy, and Fragile-X mental retardation.

The whole process of gene discovery and its use in clinical diagnosis promises to transform neurology and *psychiatry* and represents one of the greatest challenges to neuroscience. Fortunately the availability of microarrays, or "gene chips," should greatly accelerate this endeavor and provide a powerful new tool both for diagnosis and for the design of new therapies.

Apply what we know about how the brain develops.

The brain passes through specific stages of development from conception until death, and through different stages and areas of vulnerability and growth that can be either enhanced or impaired. To improve treatment for developmental disorders such as autism, attention deficit disorder, and learning disabilities, neuroscience will build a more detailed picture of brain development. Because the brain also has unique problems associated with other stages of development such as adolescence and aging, understanding how the brain changes during these periods will enable us to develop innovative treatments.

Harness the immense potential of the plasticity of the brain.

By harnessing the power of neuroplasticity—the ability of the brain to remodel and adjust itself—neuroscientists will advance treatments for degenerative neurological diseases and offer ways to improve brain function in both healthy and disease states. In the next 10 years, cell replacement therapies and the promotion of new brain cell formation will lead to new treatments for stroke, spinal cord injury, and Parkinson's disease.

Expand our understanding of what makes us uniquely human.

How does the brain work? Neuroscientists are at the point where they can ask—and begin to answer—the big questions. What are the mechanisms and underlying neural circuits that allow us to form memories, pay attention, feel and express our emotions, make decisions, use language, and foster creativity? Efforts to develop a "unified field theory" of the brain will offer great opportunities to maximize human potential.

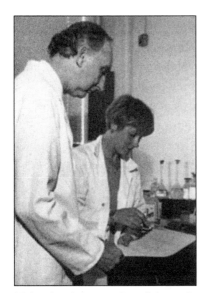

Major developments in cellular and *molecular biology* are contributing significantly to our understanding of basic brain function.

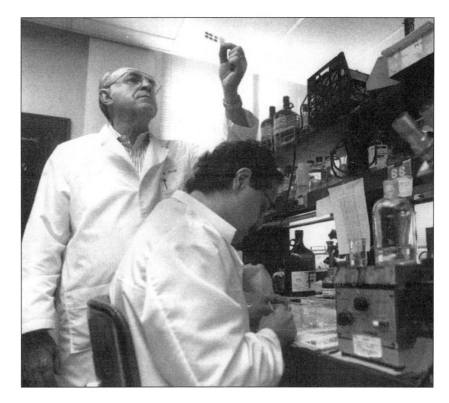

The Tools

Cell replacement

Adult nerve cells cannot replicate themselves to replace cells lost because of disease or injury. Technologies that use the ability of neural stem cells (the progenitors of neurons) to differentiate into new neurons have the potential to revolutionize the treatment of neurological disorders. Transplants of neural stem cells, currently being done on animal models, will rapidly reach human clinical trial status. How to control the development of these cells, direct them to the right place, and cause them to make the appropriate connections are all active areas of research.

Neural repair mechanisms

By using the nervous system's own repair mechanisms—in some cases, regenerating new neurons and in others restoring the wiring—the brain has the potential to "fix" itself. The ability to enhance these processes provides hope for recovery after spinal cord injury or head injuries.

Technologies that may arrest or prevent neurodegeneration

Many conditions, such as Parkinson's disease, Alzheimer's disease, Huntington's disease, and ALS, are the result of degeneration in specific populations of nerve cells in particular regions of the brain. Our present treatments, which modify the symptoms in a disease like Parkinson's disease, do not alter this progressive loss of nerve cells. Techniques that draw on our knowledge of the mechanisms of cell death are likely to offer methods to prevent neurodegeneration and, in this way, stop the progression of these diseases.

Technologies that modify genetic expression in the brain

It is possible to either enhance or block the action of specific genes in the brains of experimental animals. Mutated human genes that cause neurological diseases such as Huntington's and ALS are being used in animal models to assist in the development of new therapies to prevent neurodegeneration. Such techniques have also provided valuable information about normal processes such as development of the brain, learning, and the formation of new memories. These technologies provide an approach to the study of normal and abnormal brain processes more powerful than there has ever been available before and, in time, may be used clinically in the treatment of many brain disorders.

Advanced imaging techniques

There have been remarkable advances in imaging both the structure and the function of the brain. By developing techniques that image brain functions as quickly and accurately as the brain does, we can achieve "real-time" imaging of brain functions. These technologies will allow neuroscientists to see exactly which parts of the brain are involved as we think, learn, and experience emotions.

Electronic aids to replace nonfunctional brain pathways

In time it may be possible to bypass injured pathways in the brain. Using multi-electrode array implants and micro-computer devices—which monitor activity in the brain and translate it into signals to the spinal cord, motor nerves, or directly to muscles—we expect to be able to offer the injured hope for functional recovery.

Novel methods of drug discovery

Advances in structural biology, genomics, and computational chemistry are enabling scientists to generate unprecedented numbers of new drugs, many of which promise to be of considerable value in clinical practice. The development of new, rapid screening procedures, using "gene chips" and other high-throughput technologies, will reduce the time between the discovery of a new drug and its clinical evaluation, in some cases, from years to just a few months. ■

Chapter 5
Suggested Activities

Classroom DVD: *Dana Sourcebook of Brain Science*

Section 1: Looking Inside the Brain

Background

For the last century, scientists have been able to use the X-ray machine to examine the bony parts of the living human body, but they were not able to X-ray the living human brain. Since the 1970s, however, new computer technology has been developed that goes far beyond the capabilities of the X-ray and allows scientists to examine a living individual's functioning brain. Because of this new technology, scientists have learned a great deal about how we think, feel, and perceive.

KEY WORDS
CAT (computer-aided tomography), PET (positron emission tomography), MRI (magnetic resonance imaging), fMRI *(functional magnetic resonance imaging)*, cortex, neural

SUGGESTED RECALL QUESTIONS
1. Where is the visual cortex of the brain?

2. Where is the part of the visual cortex specific to recognizing faces? What size is it?

3. How does functional MRI, the technique used by Dr. Nancy Kanwisher in the video to image the brain, work?

4. Why is there an area of the brain dedicated to reading faces?

EXAMPLES OF DISCUSSION QUESTIONS

1. Does the new imaging technology allow scientists to "read" our minds?

2. What is the difference between the brain and the mind?

LEARN MORE ABOUT IT

View "Brain Imaging Timeline," on DVD.

Recommended Web sites:

The Whole Brain Atlas, www.med.harvard.edu/AANLIB/home.html

Digital Anatomist, http://www9.biostr.washington.edu/da.html

Classroom DVD: *Dana Sourcebook of Brain Science*

Section 2: Sports and the Brain

Background

Learning any motor skill involves a complex relationship between the body and the brain. As the body learns a particular movement through constant repetition and practice, the brain is also learning. At each new skill level, the brain stores what it has learned in a separate area while it continues to learn. Once a skill is mastered, an athlete finds ways to trigger the brain to remember what it has learned. Some athletes learn to focus solely on the activity so that the brain is not in any way distracted.

KEY WORDS

Conditioning (as in training), motor skills, coordination

SUGGESTED RECALL QUESTIONS

1. Why is it difficult to hit a baseball the first time you try?

2. How does the brain learn motor skills?

3. According to Dr. David Van Essen, what must an athlete do in order to perform successfully?

EXAMPLES OF DISCUSSION QUESTIONS

1. Is there such a thing as a born athlete?

2. What are the most important skills an athlete must develop?

LEARN MORE ABOUT IT

Read "Behind the Scenes in the Adolescent Brain," p. 34.

Recommended Web sites:

National Institute of Child Health and Human Development, www.nichd.nih.gov

National Institute of Mental Health, www.nimh.nih.gov

Classroom DVD: *Dana Sourcebook of Brain Science*

Section 3: The Broken Brain

Background

Sports are a major cause of brain injuries to children and young adults. Studies show that 7 to 10 percent of all football players will sustain at least one concussion while playing. Pat LaFontaine, a star American-born professional hockey player, had to retire from the National Hockey League after 14 years and six concussions. Multiple concussions can result in memory loss, difficulty with thinking and concentrating, and even more serious problems. Doctors and brain researchers are cautioning all athletes about the dangers of brain injuries.

KEY WORDS

Concussion, neurologist, trauma, symptomatic, migraine headaches, neuropsychological

SUGGESTED RECALL QUESTIONS

1. What is a concussion?

2. How did Pat LaFontaine's brain injuries affect his family relationships?

EXAMPLES OF DISCUSSION QUESTIONS

1. Why might an athlete, whether a professional or a student-athlete, not report problems following a head injury?

2. What can be done to help reduce the number of serious sports-related injuries?

3. If a young person suffers a concussion playing sports, should that person quit playing that sport?

LEARN MORE ABOUT IT

Read "Out of the Blue," p. 33.

Recommended Web sites:

Brain Injury Association of America, www.biausa.org

Brain Injury Services, www.braininjurysvcs.org

ThinkFirst Foundation, www.thinkfirst.org

Classroom DVD: *Dana Sourcebook of Brain Science*

Section 4: Stress and the Brain

Background

If an animal senses that it is in a stressful situation, its brain tells its body to pre-pare for a fight or to take flight. The body responds by preparing extra hor-mones to create more energy and by increasing the rate the heart pumps blood to the muscles. For most animals, this stress reaction lasts for just a short time and it saves lives. As a body is preparing for fight or flight, however, all other systems, such as physical growth and warding off diseases, are placed on hold. This means that people for whom stress has become a way of life are endanger-ing every other system in their bodies. Researchers have learned by studying primates whose systems are similar to those of human beings that those who learn to have control over their lives and are able to reduce or avoid stress live longer and healthier lives.

KEY WORDS

Fight or flight, adrenaline, hypothalamus, pituitary gland, adrenal gland, cortisol, lymphocytes, primate

SUGGESTED RECALL QUESTIONS

1. Why are zebras better equipped to deal with stress than humans? (Or, put another way, why don't zebras get ulcers?)

2. How do the brain and the body react to stress?

EXAMPLES OF DISCUSSION QUESTIONS

1. Why do some people experience more stress than others?

2. What are the major causes of stress among young people in America today?

3. What can people do to eliminate or reduce stress in their daily lives?

LEARN MORE ABOUT IT

Read "Allostatic Load Scenario 4: Too Little Is as Bad as Too Much," p. 40.
   Recommended Web sites:
      National Institute of Mental Health, www.nimh.nih.gov
      National Center for Post-Traumatic Stress Disorder, www.ncptsd.org

Classroom DVD: *Dana Sourcebook of Brain Science*

Section 5: Pain and the Brain

Background

When individuals injure any part of their bodies, the pain is transmitted to the spinal cord and on to the brain. Even if the injury is a broken bone in the foot, the pain is perceived in the brain. All of us experience acute pain when we suffer injuries, and the pain may be minor or intense. But acute pain lasts only for a while, then it subsides and eventually goes away completely when the injury has healed. Chronic pain does not go away.

KEY WORDS
Acute, chronic, sickle cell disease

SUGGESTED RECALL QUESTIONS
1. Is pain important to survival?

2. Is chronic pain a sign of personal weakness?

3. How does acute pain differ from chronic pain?

4. How does sickle cell disease cause chronic pain?

EXAMPLES OF DISCUSSION QUESTIONS
1. What are some ways people have learned to help themselves manage chronic pain?

2. Why are some people unsympathetic to another person's pain?

LEARN MORE ABOUT IT
Recommended Web sites:
American Chronic Pain Association, www.theacpa.org
American Pain Foundation, www.painfoundation.org
National Chronic Pain Outreach Association, www.chronicpain.org

Classroom DVD: *Dana Sourcebook of Brain Science*

Section 6: Depression and the Brain

Background

Millions of Americans struggle with depression, a brain disorder that researchers now know affects almost every system of the body. Depression often accompanies other diseases such as alcoholism and heart disease. Research indicates that depressed heart patients are three to four times more likely to die within six months than patients who are not depressed. Unfortunately, too many doctors and patients are unaware of the relationship between depression and other diseases, which means they fail to identify depression and fail to treat it aggressively.

KEY WORDS
Chemical imbalances, physiologic processes, syndrome, cardiologist

SUGGESTED RECALL QUESTIONS
1. **Is depression a real disease or just a convenient excuse made up by people to explain their behavior?**

2. **Does depression affect adults only?**

3. **Can depression travel through families?**

4. **How widespread is depression in the United States?**

EXAMPLES OF DISCUSSION QUESTIONS
1. **What is the difference between sadness and depression?**

2. **In what way are depression and alcoholism diseases?**

LEARN MORE ABOUT IT
Read "What Exactly Are Antidepressants?," p. 37.
   Recommended Web sites:
      Depression and Related Affective Disorders Association (DRADA), www.drada.org
      NARSAD: The Mental Health Research Association, www.narsad.org
      NAMI (National Alliance on Mental Illness), www.nami.org

Classroom DVD: *Gray Matters:* "Alcohol, Drugs, and the Brain"

Section 7

Background

Substances of abuse are a cultural phenomenon as ancient as civilization itself. Only recently, however, have scientists begun to study their effects on us and, more specifically, their effects on our brains. Why do people get addicted to drugs, tobacco, and alcohol? Why is it so hard to kick a habit? It stands to reason that since drug use is self-destructive, people would naturally avoid it. This obviously is not the case. What is not so obvious, however, is why people turn to addictive drugs. People use drugs, tobacco, and alcohol to feel good, without regard to the fact that long-term effects are very bad. Research is only now showing us how genetic and environmental factors all play a part in our susceptibility to substance addiction.

KEY WORDS
Alcoholism, dopamine, emotional memory, neurotransmitter, *physical dependence,* addiction

SUGGESTED RECALL QUESTIONS
1. What percentage of Americans smoke on a daily basis?

2. What percentage of American high school students use tobacco?

3. How many adult Americans have used an illegal drug at some point in their lives?

4. Can drug use modify your brain?

5. True or false: Nicotine is NOT an addictive substance.

6. How can alcohol abuse affect memory loss and *dementia*?

EXAMPLES OF DISCUSSION QUESTIONS
1. How do drugs give people pleasure?

2. Why do some people fall quickly into addiction, while others can experiment and then walk away?

3. Is alcoholism polygenic (i.e., involving more than one gene)?

4. Why would a person who can hold his liquor have an increased risk of becoming an alcoholic?

5. According to Dr. Alan Leshner, how can drug addiction be limited to a specific environmental context?

6. Citing Dr. Steven Hyman's statement, describe the three kinds of changes that occur in the brain as a result of long-term drug use.

LEARN MORE ABOUT IT

Read "Drugs and the Brain: (A Celebration of Alcohol)" p. 83.

Recommended Web sites:

National Institute on Alcohol Abuse and Alcoholism, www.niaaa.nih.gov

National Institute on Drug Abuse, www.nida.nih.gov

National Institute of Mental Health, www.nimh.nih.gov

Classroom DVD: *Gray Matters:* "Alcohol, Drugs, and the Brain"

Section 8

"Happy day…when all appetites controlled, all poisons subdued, there shall be neither a slave nor a drunkard on the earth."

Abraham Lincoln, 1842

Background

The allure of getting high is so powerful, so seductive, how then do we get people off drugs and keep them from relapsing? These are the questions put to modern science. Rational drug design has helped to develop effective dopamine-blocking agents. Scientists realize, however, that biological treatment mechanisms can only complement psychological and emotional therapies for those addicted to alcohol and drugs.

KEY WORDS

Relapse, *psychological dependence,* physical dependence, agonist compound, rational drug design, dopamine transport blockers, anabuse, naltrexone, methadone, Zyban

SUGGESTED RECALL QUESTIONS

1. What is methadone?

2. What recent advance in methadone treatment has occurred and why is it helpful to addicts?

3. What is naltrexone and how does it work?

4. True or false: Addiction is a complex phenomenon; therefore no single treatment can work for everyone.

5. True or false: Dealing with relapse is so difficult because the individual is often subject to the same problems that he tried to solve with drug use.

6. How do new drugs for cocaine treatment work?

EXAMPLES OF DISCUSSION QUESTIONS

1. According to Dr. Alan Leshner, what is psychological dependence as opposed to physical addiction to drugs?

2. Describe the function of methadone at the molecular level.

3. How could cocaine drugs, called dopamine transport blockers, work in dealing with cocaine addiction?

4. Pat Summerall, the host of the program, admits that he would not have quit drinking if his family had not confronted him. Would you confront a friend or family member with an addiction, or would you let him sort out his problems alone?

5. Discuss how much progress has been made in alcoholism treatment in recent years, as highlighted on the audio.

LEARN MORE ABOUT IT

Recommended Web sites:

National Institute on Alcohol Abuse and Alcoholism, www.niaaa.nih.gov

National Institute on Drug Abuse, www.nida.nih.gov

National Institute of Mental Health, www.nimh.nih.gov

Classroom DVD: *Gray Matters:* "The Arts and the Brain"

Section 9

Background

Neuroscientists and learning specialists are gaining more knowledge about how children learn and how the arts can contribute to that process. As a result of imaging technologies that permit us to "see" the neural development of the brain, we now know how important the first three years of life are to a child's cognitive development. The arts—music, drama, creative writing, and visual arts—can play a valuable role in this process by engaging a child in activities ideal in promoting the "wiring" for learning.

KEY WORDS

Cognitive development, mental schema, repetition, motor cortex, collateral benefits, meaning, and memory

SUGGESTED RECALL QUESTIONS

1. How many neurons are added every single minute to the developing brain during gestation?

2. True or false: Researchers at the University of Illinois found that rats raised with playmates, toys, and a variety of stimuli grew 25 percent more neurons than those deprived of that same stimulation.

3. How do mental schema help us make sense of the world?

EXAMPLES OF DISCUSSION QUESTIONS

1. Describe what's going on in your brain when you read music and how this might help learning in general.

2. A study conducted at Columbia University shows that students who were involved in music and the arts were much more tolerant of other people's ideas, more flexible in their approach to solving problems, and more willing to take intellectual risks. Discuss why you think this might be the case.

3. Anne Green Gilbert is head of Seattle's Creative Dance Center. She claims that "the brain only has memory when there is meaning." What do you think of this statement? Can there be memory without meaning?

4. Why is movement increasingly important as a tool for learning in today's society?

LEARN MORE ABOUT IT

Recommended Web sites:

Learning Disabilities Association of America, www.ldaamerica.org

National Coalition of Creative Arts Therapies Associations (NCCATA), www.nccata.com

Classroom DVD: *Gray Matters:* "The Arts and the Brain"

Section 10

Background

Brain scientists are exploring the neural underpinnings of art—how the arts are perceived by the brain and which cells and circuits come into play. Are artists' brains wired differently than other people's brains? How might the arts be used as therapy for people with brain injury, stroke, or Alzheimer's disease? How can the study of synesthesia open a window on brain function and cognition?

KEY WORDS

Art therapy, movement therapy, plasticity, neural networks, synesthesia and synesthetes, metronome

SUGGESTED RECALL QUESTIONS

1. What are some of the goals of arts therapy?

2. What is the potential benefit of movement therapy?

3. What is synesthesia? Name some famous synesthetes.

4. True or false: Most artists are synesthetes.

EXAMPLES OF DISCUSSION QUESTIONS

1. How can art and music therapy offer healing potential for the brain?

2. How else can art therapy help a damaged brain?

3. How common is synesthesia?

4. Dr. Vilayanur Ramachandran observes that the fusiform *gyrus* (occipitotemporal gyrus), the region of the brain responsible for seeing numbers, lies beside the part of the brain involved in seeing colors, which is itself adjacent to a primary auditory area. He considers "sloppy wiring" between these regions as a possible source of synesthesia. Why would the brain make "sloppy" connections?

LEARN MORE ABOUT IT

Recommended Web sites:

National Coalition of Creative Arts Therapies Associations (NCCATA),
www.nccata.com

National Institute of Neurological Disorders and Stroke, www.ninds.nih.gov

Chapter 6

Important Books on the Brain: An Annotated Bibliography of Fiction and Non-Fiction

The following descriptions focus on widely praised books about the brain, both scientific and literary. The selections are excerpted from articles in Cerebrum: The Dana Forum on Brain Science. Cerebrum *is now a free Web publication, with monthly articles, regular book features, letters to the editor, and a complete searchable archive of all 27 print issues from 1998–2005. To read the complete articles excerpted below, please visit* Cerebrum *online at www.dana.org.*

Authors of books who are members of the Dana Alliance for Brain Initiatives are indicated in boldface type. (For more information on the Dana Alliance, please see p. 47.)

The book descriptions found in this section are organized in the following categories:

1. The Great Brain Books, Voted by Scientists of the Dana Alliance for Brain Initiatives

2. "Ourselves To Know," Books from Scientists of the Dana Alliance

3. Great Literary Portrayals of Brain Disorders

4. The Inner Lives of Disordered Brains

5. Four Fictional Odysseys Through Life With a Disordered Brain

6. Brain Books for Budding Scientists—and All Children

1. The Great Brain Books

**Voted by Scientists of the Dana Alliance
for Brain Initiatives**

From *Cerebrum: The Dana Forum on Brain Science*,
Vol. 1, No. 1, Spring 1999 © Dana Press.

A Vision of the Brain

*By Semir Zeki. Blackwell Science Ltd. pb, 1993, $61.95.
Non-fiction.*

In this elegant and detailed analysis of how and
why we see—particularly color and motion—in a
constantly changing visual environment, Zeki
first reviews the historical twists and turns in
studying vision. He then lays out his understanding of functional specialization, integration, and
how our conscious perception of what we see
arises in the brain.

An Unquiet Mind: A Memoir of Moods and Madness

*By Kay Redfield Jamison. Vintage pb, 1997, $13.95.
(Originally published in hardcover by Knopf, 1995.)
Non-fiction.*

Jamison, professor of psychiatry at Johns Hopkins
University, suffers from manic depression. Here,
she reveals how this illness can woo its victims
with exalted flights of mind so exhilarating that
taking lithium to save their sanity can become an
agonizing decision. Jamison makes that issue real
for us—in personal, poetic, and scientific terms—
as no other writer ever has.

Awakenings

*By Oliver Sacks. Vintage pb, 1999, $15.95. (Originally
published in hardcover by Doubleday, 1974.) $15.00.
Non-fiction.*

This Sacks classic is the account of victims of a
decades-long sleeping sickness (encephalitis
lethargica) who awaken to a new life after being
treated with the drug L-dopa. Here, Sacks is able
to enter into the world of someone with a neurological disease and help us understand both our
common humanity and the medical science.

Brain, Mind, and Behavior

*By Floyd Bloom and Arlyne Lazerson. Worth Publishers
pb, 2000, $78.00. (Originally published in hardcover by
W.H. Freeman, 1984.) Non-fiction.*

Written to accompany a PBS-TV series, *Brain,
Mind, and Behavior* systematically moves from
monoamine transmitters to thinking and consciousness. The book is eminently readable, and
it addresses subtle controversies and questions
in research.

Bright Air, Brilliant Fire: On the Matter of the Mind

*By Gerald M. Edelman. Basic Books pb, 1993, $22.00.
(Originally published in hardcover by Basic Books,
1992.) Non-fiction.*

A Nobel laureate presents his complex and revo-
lutionary vision of how evolution has led from
simple cells to the intricate biology of our
brains—and, in Edelman's view, our extraordinary minds and unique human consciousness.

Descartes' Error: Emotion, Reason, and the Human Brain

*By Antonio R. Damasio. Penguin pb, 2005, $15.00.
(Originally published in hardcover by G.P. Putnam's
Sons, 1994.) Non-fiction.*

The first modern European philosopher, René
Descartes, saw mind and body as fundamentally
separate. The idea infected Western thought with
the premise that rationality and feeling, the mental and the biological, don't mix. Damasio challenges that dualism root and branch, marshaling
evidence from basic and clinical research and
interpreting it with rare philosophical acuity.

Drugs and the Brain

*By Solomon H. Snyder. Scientific American Library pb,
1996, $24.95. (Originally published in hardcover by
Scientific American Books, Inc., 1986.) Non-fiction.*

Snyder tells the story of brain research from the
viewpoint of brain chemistry and pharmacologi-
cal agents (some known over thousands of years)
and what they reveal about our brains. The 1996
paperback updates the story with molecular biology, gene cloning, and discovery of neurotransmitter receptors, as well as the practical story of

new drugs such as Prozac for depression and clozapine for schizophrenia.

Essentials of Neural Science and Behavior

Edited by **Eric Kandel,** *James Schwartz, and Thomas Jessell. McGraw-Hill/Appleton & Lange, 1995, $79.95. Non-fiction.*

This is a textbook for undergraduates with some biology experience. Three primary authors, all at Columbia University, are joined by a dozen more to present the subject—from neuron to memory—with many illustrations, all technical, and appropriate mathematical formulas and models of compounds.

Evolving Brains

By John Morgan Allman. Scientific American Library pb, 2000, $22.95. (Originally published in hardcover by W.H. Freeman, 1999.) Non-fiction.

A distinguished contributor in his own right to brain research on vision, Allman brings a rare combination of neuroscience, evolutionary biology, and developmental biology to his work. *Evolving Brains* is a fascinating account of the uncanny, unconscious genius of evolution brilliantly improvising the brain in response to the needs of the gut, the blood, the hunt, and, always, the next generation.

Eye and Brain: The Psychology of Seeing

By Richard L. Gregory. Princeton University Press pb, 1997, $22.95. (Originally published in hardcover by Weidenfeld & Nicolson, 1966.) Non-fiction.

Gregory has a special slant: approaching vision through the analysis and categorization of visual illusions. In this, he is a pioneer, making the book unique (not to mention fascinating), with visual illusions to illustrate each chapter and to make you realize that deep mysteries remain.

Eye, Brain, and Vision

By **David H. Hubel.** *Scientific American Library pb, 1995, $32.95. (Originally published in hardcover by W.H. Freeman, 1988.) Non-fiction.*

For their role in the knowledge revolution surrounding vision, Hubel and **Torsten N. Wiesel**

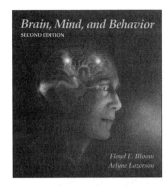
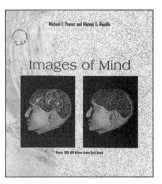
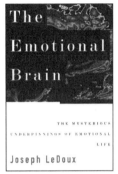
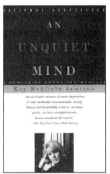

received a Nobel Prize in 1981. Here Hubel tells the story for readers, he says, with scientific training but not biology expertise. Trained or not, readers who like science—and how a great scientist thinks—will enjoy this book.

Galen's Prophecy: Temperament in Human Nature

By **Jerome Kagan.** *Westview Press pb, 1998, $38.00. (Originally published in hardcover by Basic Books, 1994.) Non-fiction.*

Psychologist Jerome Kagan takes a perceptive look at what research into infant and child development can teach us about human nature, in particular the biological influences on temperament.

How the Mind Works

By Steven Pinker. W.W. Norton pb, 1999, $17.95. (Originally published in hardcover by W.W. Norton, 1997.) Non-fiction.

Pinker attempts to explain the brain's natural ability to perform feats that even the most sophisticated computer hardware would find impossible. He also explores how the mind thinks, reasons, falls in love, and develops family bonds.

Images of Mind

*By **Michael I. Posner** and **Marcus Raichle**. W.H. Freeman pb, 1997, $19.95. (Originally published in hardcover by Scientific American Library, 1994.) Non-fiction.*

This volume—by a foremost cognitive psychologist (Posner) and a pioneer of positron emission tomography (Raichle)—is not just a book on imaging; it is also a general brain book. Chapters deal with mental images, interpreting words, mental operations, attention, brain development, and mental disorders. Visuals, including brain scans, are generous, but so is the lucid text.

Listening to Prozac: A Psychiatrist Explores Antidepressant Drugs and the Remaking of the Self

By Peter D. Kramer. Penguin pb, 1997, $16.00. (Originally published in hardcover by Viking Penguin, 1993.) Non-fiction.

If Prozac transforms personalities of relatively healthy patients, what does this mean for our view of psychiatry? Mental illness? Biology as destiny? In his book, Kramer raises and deliberatively deepens the issues.

Mapping Fate: A Memoir of Family, Risk, and Genetic Research

By Alice Wexler. University of California Press pb, 1996, $19.95. (Originally published in hardcover by Crown, 1995.) Non-fiction.

In *Mapping Fate*, Wexler skillfully interweaves the heartbreaking story of her family's odyssey with Huntington's disease—which killed her mother—and the dramatic, suspenseful, and eventually triumphant scientific search for the Huntington's gene, spearheaded by her sister and her father.

Memory and Brain

*By **Larry R. Squire**. Oxford University Press pb, 1987, $31.95. (Originally published in hardcover by Oxford University Press, 1987.) Non-fiction.*

Looking back at two decades of productive research on memory, Squire sets out to integrate the work of psychologists and neurobiologists into a coherent account of the nature of memory: synaptic changes, storage, learning, information processing, and types of memory.

Molecules and Mental Illness

By Samuel H. Barondes. W.H. Freeman pb, 1999, $19.95. (Originally published in hardcover by Scientific American Library, 1993.) Non-fiction.

This book teaches molecular biology while telling the story of biological psychiatry. Barondes guides you through heredity, molecular genetics, cellular neuroscience, and psychopharmacology with fascinating sidelights and fine Scientific American Library illustrations while creating vivid portraits of manic-depressive illness, major depression, schizophrenia, and disabling fears and compulsions.

Mood Genes: Hunting for Origins of Mania and Depression

By Samuel H. Barondes. Oxford University Press pb, 1999, $22.00. (Originally published in hardcover by W.H. Freeman, 1998.) Non-fiction.

The search is on for genes affecting complex mental disorders and, in particular, those underlying mania and depression using linkage studies of families in Costa Rica. Barondes, a gene hunter, tells this story in terms of sufferers and scientists, bringing out the excitement, complexity, and controversies.

Neuronal Man: The Biology of Mind

By Jean-Pierre Changeux. Princeton University Press pb, 1997, $24.95. (Originally published in hardcover by Fayard, 1983.) Non-fiction.

In this book, Changeux devotes more than the usual attention to history and to cross-species comparisons that probe why human brains are so relatively capable. Unlike some introductions to the brain, *Neuronal Man* has few illustrations. It does, however, have a glossary and an extensive bibliography.

Recollections of My Life

By Santiago Ramón y Cajal. MIT Press pb, 1989, $32.00. (Originally published 1901–1917 in Madrid.) Non-fiction.

One "founder" of neuroscience is Ramón y Cajal, a Spanish histologist born in 1852 whose massive writings and superb drawings are still the most cited sources on the nervous system. *Recollections* is the story not only of his methods and chief discoveries, but of the astonishing life that began with boyhood rebellions and rose to every triumph, including the Nobel Prize (with Camillo Golgi) in 1906.

Searching for Memory: The Brain, the Mind, and the Past

By Daniel L. Schacter. Basic Books pb, 1997, $18.95. (Originally published in hardcover by Basic Books, 1996.) Non-fiction.

Schacter, chairman of psychology at Harvard, tells the story that brain research has found to explain the multiple, complex systems that underlie memory. We learn that with memory's power comes fragility, limitations seen not only in disease and aging but also in explosive issues such as "recovered memories" of child abuse that have put innocent teachers in prison.

The Astonishing Hypothesis: The Scientific Search for the Soul

By Francis Crick. Scribner pb, 1995, $15.00. (Originally published in hardcover by Scribner, 1994.) Non-fiction.

The "astonishing hypothesis" is that "all aspects of the brain's behavior are due to the activities of neurons" (that's *all*, including lofty aspects once called "soul"). Confronting religious explanations head-on, Crick's challenge is to make real to us what it would mean to provide a complete explanation of awareness solely in neural terms.

The Broken Brain: The Biological Revolution in Psychiatry

By Nancy Andreasen. HarperPerennial pb, 1985, $15.95. (Originally published in hardcover by Harper & Row, 1984.) Non-fiction.

Andreasen, a distinguished psychiatrist, introduces this book with chapters on the history of mental illness, the brain, the four major syndromes, diagnosis, treatment, and research. Many authors claim to write for laymen; Andreasen, a former English teacher, really does. Her subtext is that mental illness is a disease, no more shameful than cancer.

The Emotional Brain: The Mysterious Underpinnings of Emotional Life

By Joseph LeDoux. Touchstone pb, 1998, $14.00. (Originally published in hardcover by Simon & Schuster, 1996.) Non-fiction.

The Emotional Brain reasons its way through questions about the nature of emotions, conservation of emotional systems across species, conscious and unconscious emotional responses, and the relationship between feelings and emotions.

The History of Neuroscience in Autobiography, Vols. 1 and 2

Edited by Larry R. Squire. Society for Neuroscience, 1996 and 1998. Vol. I: $63.95; Vol. II: $65.95. Non-fiction.

As president of the Society for Neuroscience, Squire, a pioneer of memory research, conceived of this series and edited both volumes. Well-known neuroscientists from America and Europe contributed, with pieces running from fairly autobiographical (Herbert H. Jasper) to mostly scientific (Sir Bernard Katz). There are good photographs of each scientist.

The Language Instinct: How the Mind Creates Language

By Steven Pinker. HarperPerennial pb, 1995, $15.00. (Originally published in hardcover by William Morrow, 1994.) Non-fiction.

Steven Pinker, a psychologist, turns a phenomenon that most of us take for granted—language—into a wonder and mystery that, he proposes, is at the heart of human development. Disputing the theory that language is a cultural construct, he argues that it is ingrained, an "instinct," as hardwired in humans as making a web is in spiders. Includes notes and a brief glossary.

The Longevity Strategy: How to Live to 100 Using the Brain-Body Connection

By David Mahoney and Richard Restak. Foreword by William Safire. John Wiley & Sons, Inc., and Dana Press pb, 1999, $14.95. (Originally published in hardcover by John Wiley & Sons, Inc., and Dana Press, 1998.) Non-fiction.

Mahoney, the business executive and philanthropist who was chairman of the Dana Alliance for

Brain Initiatives, teamed up with the neurologist and neuropsychiatrist Restak for this road map to a healthy longevity. Includes 31 practical, research-based tactics for maintaining cognitive and emotional well-being, physical health, and financial stability through the life span.

The Man Who Mistook His Wife for a Hat and Other Clinical Tales
By Oliver Sacks. Touchstone pb, 1998, $14.00. (Originally published in hardcover by Simon & Schuster, 1970.) Non-fiction.

Patients with lesions and disorders have been a crucial window on the brain for neuroscientists. In this famous book. Sacks presents a series of such case studies, from Korsakov's syndrome, with its devastation of memory, to Tourette's syndrome, with its explosion of mental energy, in portraits that are profoundly revelatory and full of compassion for the afflicted individuals.

The Organization of Behavior: A Neuropsychological Theory
By Donald O. Hebb. Lawrence Erlbaum Associates, 2002, $45.00. (Originally published by John Wiley & Sons, Inc., 1949.) Non-fiction.

Hebb, a pioneering psychologist at the University of Montreal, is remembered most of all for his statement of the principle that coactivation of neurons is required to strengthen the synaptic connection. This is cited in most accounts of learning theory and is called "Hebb's Rule." *The Organization of Behavior* was Hebb's culminating report to the world on his work and is still a classic.

The Placebo Effect: An Interdisciplinary Exploration
Edited by Anne Harrington. Harvard University Press pb, 1999, $24.50. (Originally published in hardcover by Harvard University Press, 1997.) Non-fiction.

An insightful collection of essays and dialogues that looks at placebos from viewpoints as diverse as neuropharmacology and anthropology, molecular biology and religion. Contributors place placebos at the intersection of biology and culture, with much to teach us about the interaction of our minds and bodies.

The Principles of Psychology
By William James. Dover Publications pb, 2 vols., 1950, $16.95/volume. (Originally published in hardcover by Henry Holt, 1890.) Non-fiction.

Stream of thought, consciousness of self, attention, conception, perception of time, memory: James analyzed, categorized, and conceptualized each aspect of mental life. Much remains valid—and not infrequently used as the starting point of discussions today—because James knew and honored the difference between observation and interpretation.

The Rediscovery of the Mind
By John R. Searle. MIT Press pb, 1992, $25.00. (Originally published in hardcover by MIT Press, 1992.) Non-fiction.

Having rejected materialism and dualism, and having admitted consciousness to the natural world, Searle analyzes its nature. His arguments are cogent, as is his dissection of materialism, which irks cognitive scientists whose investigations avoid all reference to mental life. But to study the brain while dismissing consciousness, says Searle, is like studying biology while explaining away the inconvenient emergence of life.

Why Zebras Don't Get Ulcers: The Acclaimed Guide to Stress, Stress-Related Diseases, and Coping, Third Edition
By Robert M. Sapolsky. Owl Books pb, 2004, $16.00. (Originally published in hardcover by W.H. Freeman, 1993.) Non-fiction.

Evolution of the fight-or-flight mechanism that, in a burst of physiological fireworks, can save a zebra from a lion, is often turned on—and left on—by the psychological and social stressors in our lives. Then the sympathetic nervous system's response to "danger" becomes the problem. Sapolsky explains all this, writing about glucocorticoids and insulin secretion with wit and charm.

2. "Ourselves to Know"

Books from Scientists of the Dana Alliance
From *Cerebrum: The Dana Forum on Brain Science,*
Vol. 6, No. 2, Spring 2004 © Dana Press.

A Passion for DNA: Genes, Genomes, and Society

*By **James D. Watson**. Cold Spring Harbor Laboratory Press pb, 2001, $15.00. (Originally published in hardcover by Cold Spring Harbor Laboratory Press, 2000.) Non-fiction.*

A collection of Watson's essays in which he commented on scientific advances that were taking place during his 30 years as director and later president of the Cold Spring Harbor Laboratory, one of the world's foremost in molecular biology.

A Universe of Consciousness: How Matter Becomes Imagination

*By **Gerald Edelman** and Giulio Tononi. Basic Books pb, 2001, $18.00. (Originally published in hardcover by Basic Books, 2000.) Non-fiction.*

Nobel laureate Edelman has not just pondered the problem of consciousness; for some 25 years, he has conducted scientific research on it, publishing a string of books. *A Universe of Consciousness,* co-authored with neurobiologist Tononi, sums up and interprets these investigations in "the main outlines of a solution to the problem of consciousness."

Base Instincts: What Makes Killers Kill?

*By **Jonathan Pincus**. W.W. Norton pb, 2002, $14.95. (Originally published in hardcover by Diane Publishing Co., 2001.) Non-fiction.*

A 25-year study of 150 murderers on death row, in locked psychiatric wards, and in prisons, reveals "a strong tie between violent behavior and neurological abnormalities, paranoid thoughts, and the experience of severe, prolonged, physical abuse," according to the author.

Brain-Wise: Studies in Neurophilosophy

*By **Patricia Smith Churchland**. MIT Press pb, 2002, $28.00. (Originally published in hardcover by MIT Press, 2002.) Non-fiction.*

Framed as philosophy, not neuroscience, *Brain-Wise* is organized around traditional domains of philosophy, such as metaphysics, epistemology, free will, and religion. Its defining thesis is that if philosophers pose old philosophical problems (the nature of mind, the nature of self, the nature of learning) in light of discoveries in brain and cognitive science, they will at last make genuine progress.

Brave New Brain: Conquering Mental Illness in the Era of the Genome

*By **Nancy Andreasen**. Oxford University Press pb, 2004, $17.95. (Originally published in hardcover by Oxford University Press, 2001.) Non-fiction.*

Describes progress over a decade or more in understanding the chief categories of mental illness (schizophrenia, dementia, mood disorders, and anxiety disorders), how treatments have changed, especially in light of understanding the genetics of illness, and what lies ahead. Includes a mini-tutorial on neuroscience and molecular genetics, a review of mental illnesses, and comments on what it all means in social and economic terms.

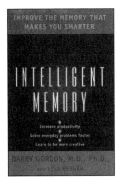
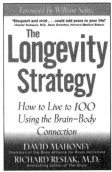
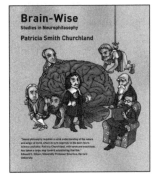
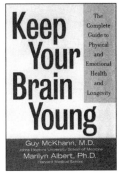

DNA: The Secret of Life

*By **James D. Watson,** with Andrew Berry. Alfred A. Knopf pb, 2004, $24.95. (Originally published in hardcover by Alfred A. Knopf, 2003.) Non-fiction.*

A big book with full-color illustrations that tells the story of DNA. Not just a coffee-table book, the consensus among scientists is that it is vintage Watson in style and intellectual level, giving him the opportunity to comment on the significance of molecular biology over half a century and where we might be going with it.

Genes, Girls, and Gamow: After the Double Helix

*By **James D. Watson.** Vintage pb, 2003, $14.00. (Originally published in hardcover by Alfred A. Knopf, 2002.) Non-fiction.*

Far and away his most personal book, *Genes, Girls, and Gamow* is the story of what Watson did following his co-discovery, with Francis Crick, of the structure of DNA. The book tells how, as a world-famous scientist at 25, Watson spent his time studying ribonucleic acid (RNA) to understand how genes encode proteins, and how he went about finding himself a wife.

I of the Vortex: From Neurons to Self

*By **Rodolfo Llinas.** MIT Press pb, 2002, $19.95. (Originally published in hardcover by MIT Press, 2001.) Non-fiction.*

Described by the author as "a personal view of neuroscience" from the perspective of "a single-cell physiologist interested in neuronal integration and synaptic transmission." What emerges in this book is a sweeping integration of this cell-level perspective with insights at levels from the molecular to the technologic-social. The result is a new theory of the nature of mind, which, according to Llinas, evolved to enable living creatures to succeed in their environment by being able to predict—the ultimate brain function.

Intelligent Memory: Improve Your Memory No Matter What Your Age

*By **Barry Gordon** and Lisa Berger. Penguin, 2005, $14.00. (Originally published in hardcover by Viking Adult, 2003.) Non-fiction.*

Outlines ways to develop the mental processes that direct what the authors term "intelligent memory," the very engine which powers our intelligence. Sharpening this tool makes us able to think creatively, anticipate problems, and infer solutions rapidly. Includes an exploration of mental processes and a series of memory exercises and quizzes that are challenging and fun.

Keep Your Brain Young: The Complete Guide to Physical and Emotional Health and Longevity

*By **Guy McKhann** and **Marilyn Albert.** John Wiley & Sons, Inc./Dana Press pb, 2003, $15.95. (Originally published in hardcover by John Wiley & Sons, Inc. and Dana Press, 2002.) Non-fiction.*

A guide to what you can expect in every area of life that involves the brain as you move past 50: memory, nutrition, sleep, depression, alcohol, pain, sexual function, vision and other senses, and the serious illnesses like Alzheimer's disease that affect the brain in older age. The book moves from the wisdom of the seasoned physician to the latest in research discoveries.

Liars, Lovers, and Heroes: What the New Brain Science Reveals About How We Become Who We Are

*By **Steven R. Quartz** and **Terrence Sejnowski.** Harper pb, 2003, $14.95. (Originally published in hardcover by William Morrow, 2002.) Non-fiction.*

Liars, Lovers, and Heroes calls on recent advances in brain imaging, computer modeling, and genetics as well as historical and contemporary theories of philosophy, psychology, politics, and sociology to answer questions like: Who are we? Why do we love and hate? Why do we sometimes lay down our lives for others? Why do we sometimes kill? On a range of topics, including sex, learning, violence, and happiness, the authors provide an accessible account of how our brains and world engage, excite, and alter each other.

Looking for Spinoza: Joy, Sorrow, and the Feeling Brain

*By **Antonio Damasio**. Harvest Books pb, 2003, $15.00. (Originally published in hardcover by Harcourt, Inc., 2003.) Non-fiction.*

Examines the role in human existence of feelings and the emotions that underlie feelings (an important distinction for Damasio). Damasio shares his rediscovery of the 17th-century Dutch philosopher Benedict Spinoza whose *Ethics* defied the life-and-death power of religion in his era in postulating the inseparability of mind and body. *Looking for Spinoza* is a complete work of philosophy as well as science, rooting a modern-day philosophy of human nature, the good life, and the just society in the discoveries of brain science.

Matter of Mind: A Neurologist's View of Brain-Behavior Relationships

*By **Kenneth M. Heilman**. Oxford University Press, 2002, $39.95. Non-fiction.*

By studying how mind and behavior are affected by brain injury, scientists since the Greek physician Hippocrates have mapped the brain. In this book, Heilman tells how lesions in the brain change—often in astonishing ways—language, emotion, attention, self-awareness, memory, cognitive-motor skills, sensory perception, and intention.

Memory and Emotion: The Making of Lasting Memories

*By **James McGaugh**. Columbia University Press, 2003, $27.50. Non-fiction.*

McGaugh, professor of neurobiology and behavior at the University of California, Irvine, and pioneer in memory research, discusses the history of memory research, recent major discoveries, the molecular biological processes underlying formation of long-term memories, new ideas about post-traumatic stress disorder (PTSD), and more in an engaging and personable style.

Mozart's Brain and the Fighter Pilot: Unleashing Your Brain's Potential

*By **Richard Restak**. Three Rivers Press pb, 2002, $12.00. (Originally published in hardcover by Harmony Books, 2001.) Non-fiction.*

Can we make ourselves smarter? Restak suggests in this book that a good grasp of how your brain works can even make you more intelligent. With more that 20 exercises intended to improve memory, creativity, and concentration by increasing neural linkages, this best-selling guide promises to enhance your cognitive capabilities now and into old age.

Mysteries of the Mind

*By **Richard Restak**. National Geographic, 2000, $35.00. Non-fiction.*

Mysteries of the Mind takes readers on a tour of the brain, using drawings and illustrations to explore its structure and operation, particularly in sleep, memory, and emotion.

Overcoming Dyslexia: A New and Complete Science-Based Program for Reading Problems at Any Level

*By **Sally Shaywitz**. Vintage pb, 2005, $15.95. (Originally published in hardcover by Alfred A. Knopf, 2003.) Non-fiction.*

A trusted authority on dyslexia for over 20 years, Shaywitz provides a comprehensive source of information and guidance, answering questions she has heard in years on the lecture circuit. All three sections of the book—on the nature of dyslexia, its diagnosis, and how to overcome it—are enlivened with personal stories from Shaywitz's work with students, teachers, and parents.

Parkinson's Disease: A Complete Guide for Patients and Families

*By **William J. Weiner, Lisa M. Shulman, and **Anthony E. Lang**. Johns Hopkins University Press pb, 2001, $20.95. (Originally published in hardcover by Johns Hopkins University Press, 2001.) Non-fiction.*

A straightforward, comprehensive guide to living with Parkinson's disease as long and healthfully as possible. Treatments developed over the past three decades make prospects for the patient far better but also offer many options to be considered. Issues such as these and others are addressed by the authors in well-organized sections that are written in clear, unaffected prose.

Striking Back at Stroke: A Doctor-Patient Journal

*By Cleo Hutton and **Louis Caplan**. Dana Press, 2003, $27.00. Non-fiction.*

In *Striking Back at Stroke*, Hutton's personal narrative of her stroke and rehabilitation alternate with commentary by Caplan, a professor of neurology who is a leading clinical researcher on stroke. The result is a vivid yet informed account, immediate but thoughtful about how a patient and modern medical science together fought back against a "brain attack." *(See excerpt, p. 35.)*

Surprise, Uncertainty and Mental Structures

*By **Jerome Kagan**. Harvard University Press, 2002, $37.50. Non-fiction.*

In this book, Kagan asks whether any single type of mental operation (for example, behavioral conditioning, imagery, or concepts in words) can account for the wide diversity of human behavior, thought, and emotion. He argues for the existence of at least two basically different modes of mental operation, which he calls "schemata" (picturing things) and "semantic networks" (putting things in words), and shows how this distinction illuminates thinking about psychological development, creativity, and personality measurement and theory.

Synaptic Self: How Our Brains Become Who We Are

*By **Joseph LeDoux**. Penguin pb, 2003, $16.00. (Originally published in hardcover by Viking Adult, 2002.) Non-fiction.*

LeDoux is interested here in examining how our brains—in particular the inconceivably complex "connectivity" of brain cells at many levels—make possible who we are. To this end, *Synaptic Self* turns to a vast array of brain science, including the research that LeDoux reported in *The Emotional Brain* (1996). His basic claim: "The bottom-line point of this book is, you are your synapses."

The Dana Guide to Brain Health

Floyd E. Bloom, M. Flint Beal, and David J. Kupfer, Editors. Foreword by William Safire. Free Press, 2003, $45.00. Non-fiction. (Paperback edition with CD-ROM coming Fall 2006.)

The first comprehensive home reference book about the brain, how it works when it is healthy, and what happens when things go wrong. Includes contributions from 104 top doctors and researchers and an extended section on brain and nervous system disorders that covers more than 70 neurological and emotional conditions and how they are diagnosed and treated. *(See excerpt, p. 34.)*

The Dying of Enoch Wallace: Life, Death, and the Changing Brain

*By **Ira Black**. McGraw-Hill, 2001, $24.95. Non-fiction.*

This book presents a new model for explaining neuroscience to the lay reader. Black tells two stories simultaneously, the history of neuroscience in the 20th century and the story of an investment banker, Enoch Wallace, who is diagnosed with Alzheimer's disease and who suffers the inevitable cognitive decline.

The End of Stress as We Know It

*By **Bruce McEwen** with Elizabeth N. Lasley. Dana Press/Joseph Henry Press pb, 2004, $19.95. (Originally published in hardcover by Dana Press/Joseph Henry Press, 2002.) Non-fiction.*

If the stress reaction, known as fight-or-flight, evolved to help us in emergencies, why does it also cause so much harm? Authors McEwen and Lasley address this paradox by mapping the relationship between brain function and stress responses and tell us how we can make ourselves more resilient to stress. *(See excerpt, p. 40.)*

The New Brain: How the Modern Age Is Rewiring Your Mind

*By **Richard Restak**. Rodale Press pb, 2004, $14.95. (Originally published in hardcover by Rodale Press, 2003.) Non-fiction.*

In this book, Restak looks at the progress brain science has made in just the past two decades. In this era of The New Brain, we have available the latest imaging techniques to enable us to watch the brain as it thinks, decides, and acts. Restak contends that other new technologies will become important in shaping the further evolution of our brains.

The Secret Life of the Brain
By Richard Restak. Joseph Henry Press/Dana Press, 2001, $35.00. Non-fiction.

A companion volume to the Emmy-winning PBS series of the same name. Extending beyond the television series, Restak draws on interviews and clinical research to explore life's five stages of brain development, emphasizing the brain's remarkable resilience.

The Seven Sins of Memory (How the Mind Forgets and Remembers)
By Daniel Schacter. Houghton Mifflin pb, 2002, $14.00. (Originally published in hardcover by Houghton Mifflin, 2001.) Non-fiction.

Schacter's angle here is "the nature of memory's imperfections" and how we can reduce or avoid the harm they do. He calls his schema for these imperfections the "seven sins of memory": transience, absent-mindedness, blocking, misattribution, suggestibility, bias, and persistence. These transgressions, he argues, are excesses of otherwise adaptive, useful features of our minds.

Understanding Depression: What We Know and What You Can Do About It
By J. Raymond DePaulo, Jr. and Lesley Alan Horvitz. Foreword by Kay Redfield Jamison. John Wiley & Sons Inc., and Dana Press pb, 2003, $15.95. (Originally published in hardcover by John Wiley & Sons Inc., and Dana Press, 2002.) Non-fiction.

A leading authority on depression explains how people can recognize depression in themselves or in loved ones, presents the many factors that cause people to become depressed, and discusses the proliferating options for treatment. DePaulo also presents a similar analysis of the symptoms and causes of bipolar disorder (manic depressive illness). He calls on the latest brain research to explain what doctors and researchers really know about these debilitating diseases. *(See excerpt, p. 37.)*

Vision and Art: The Biology of Seeing
By Margaret Livingstone. Harry N. Abrams, Inc., 2002, $45.00. Non-fiction.

In an easy-to-follow format, Livingstone, a neurobiologist at Harvard and vision researcher for over two decades, begins with basic reviews of the principles of light and the structure of the vertebrate eye. She then explains how we process color and luminance (lightness), the visual "what and where" system, and other aspects of how we see. She then applies this knowledge to well-known works of art. For example, how do acuity and spatial resolution explain why da Vinci's *Mona Lisa* has such a mysterious smile?

Why We See What We Do: An Empirical Theory of Vision
By Dale Purves and R. Beau Lotto. Sinauer Associates, Inc., pb, 2003, $49.95. Non-fiction.

Drawing on much of their own individual research, authors Purves and Lotto propose a new theory of vision according to which retinal stimuli trigger a reflex response in our brains. What we experience when we see is shaped by what this stimulus has come to signify in the past. Includes chapter introductions and summaries, a complete glossary, and over 100 diagrams.

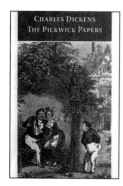
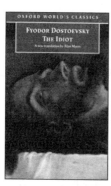
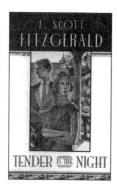
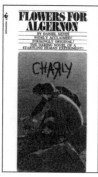
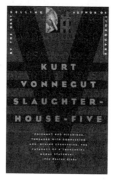

3. Great Literary Portrayals of Brain Disorders

By Marcia Clendenen and Dick Riley
Originally published as "Madness in Good Company: Great Literary Portrayals of Brain Disorders."
From *Cerebrum: The Dana Forum on Brain Science,* Vol. 2, No. 3, Summer 2000 © Dana Press.

To put these works in a current clinical context, the authors have compared the characteristics and behavior of the characters to the symptoms described in the 1994 edition of the American Psychiatric Association's *Diagnostic and Statistical Manual of Mental Disorders,* or *DSM-IV,* the standard descriptive and cataloging text for mental ailments.

"A Hunger Artist"
By Franz Kafka. Twisted Spoon Press, 1996, $13.50. (Originally published in 1924.) Fiction.
"During these last decades the interest in professional fasting has markedly diminished," begins Franz Kafka in his short story "A Hunger Artist." Those who willingly starve themselves are defined by the *DSM-IV* as having anorexia nervosa. Certainly the hunger artist exhibits behaviors mentioned in the *DSM*, including "depressive symptoms such as depressed mood, social withdrawal, irritability, insomnia."

Flowers for Algernon
By Daniel Keyes. HarcourtBrace pb, 2004, $7.99. (Originally published in 1966.) Fiction.
Charlie Gordon is a 32-year-old mentally retarded man who becomes a genius, thanks to a sketchily described new treatment, only to have the process reverse itself. Charlie himself narrates his transformation from a bakery janitor with an intelligence quotient of 68 to a man with an "intelligence that can't really be calculated." The *DSM-IV* lists both biological and psychosocial factors as potential causes of mental retardation.

Junky
By William S. Burroughs. Penguin pb, 2003, $14.00. (Originally published in 1953.) Fiction.
"Junk is not a kick. It is a way of life," says Burroughs in his "memoir of a life of addiction." He omits few of the *DSM-IV* signs of the substance abuser, including "failure to fulfill major role obligations at work, school, or home," and "continued substance use despite having persistent or recurrent…problems caused or exacerbated by the effects of the substance."

Mrs. Dalloway
By Virginia Woolf. Harvest Books, 1990, $12.00. (Originally published in 1925.) Fiction.
Mrs. Dalloway takes us through one day in the life of Clarissa Dalloway, an upper-class Englishwoman. Her life is contrasted with the tragic story of another major character, Septimus Warren Smith. The novel is set after the end of World War I. Smith had served in the war and suffers from "shell shock," the term then applied to post-traumatic stress disorder.

"Silent Snow, Secret Snow"
By Conrad Aiken. Creative Company, 1983. (Originally published in 1934. Out of print. Used copies available in bookstores or online.) Fiction.
This short story portrays a 12-year-old boy slipping into an autistic state. Paul avoids the doctor's eyes ("marked impairment in the use of multiple nonverbal behaviors such as eye-to-eye

gaze" is one of the DSM's criteria for autism) or else stares, preoccupied with the light in his pupils. Finally he smiles at the secret snow filling the corners of the room.

Slaughterhouse-Five
By Kurt Vonnegut. Dial Press pb, 1999, $14.00. (Originally published in 1969.) Fiction.
This novel tells in a nonlinear narrative of the capture of a young soldier, Billy Pilgrim, and his survival in a meat locker deep below the place where the prisoners are billeted. "Recurrent and intrusive distressing recollections," a classic symptom of post-traumatic stress disorder (PTSD), according to the *DSM-IV*, could well describe this novel.

Tender Is the Night
By F. Scott Fitzgerald. Scribner pb, 1995, $13.00. (Originally published in 1934.) Fiction.
In *Tender Is the Night,* we observe the tumultuous relationship between Nicole, once diagnosed as schizophrenic, and Dick Diver, who undergoes an alcoholic, downward spiral and professional ruin. Fitzgerald suffered from alcoholism; his wife, Zelda, was diagnosed as schizophrenic and hospitalized. *Tender Is the Night* was the last novel Fitzgerald completed.

The Accidental Tourist
By Anne Tyler. Ballantine pb, 2002, $14.95. (Originally published in 1985.) Fiction.
Macon Levy's son has been senselessly murdered. Macon's reaction is to create a world of routines, rituals, and dependable habits that hold his grief at bay. The *DSM-IV* describes obsessive-compulsive disorder as manifesting repetitive behaviors that a person feels driven to perform, behaviors that are aimed—however unrealistically—at preventing or reducing distress or at forestalling some dreaded event or situation.

The Bell Jar
By Sylvia Plath. HarperPerrenial pb, 2005, $13.95. (Originally published in 1963.) Fiction.
Esther Greenwood fits many of the *DSM-IV* criteria for depressive personality disorder. She begins electroshock therapy, but her obsession with thoughts of death worsens. For all its grim subject matter, *The Bell Jar* is full of humor, particularly in its opening passages, and has been described as a female version of the male adolescent rite-of-passage novel *A Catcher in the Rye.*

The Eden Express
By Mark Vonnegut. Seven Stories Press pb, 2004, $13.95. (Originally published in 1975.) Non-fiction.
This is an autobiographical account of Vonnegut's descent into madness, diagnosed at the time (1970) as schizophrenia. His first psychotic break occurs on a trip and consists of episodes of uncontrolled crying, shaking, and social blunders. This combination of depressive and manic episodes would probably be attributed today to bipolar disorder rather than schizophrenia.

The Idiot
By Fyodor Dostoevsky. Vintage pb, 2003, $12.95. (Originally published in 1869.) Fiction.
Born in 1821, Dostoevsky became linked with the forces of political reform in Russia. He and a group of friends were arrested for political activity, tried, and sentenced to death. In a dreadful charade, with Dostoevsky already on the scaffold, the sentence was commuted and he was sent to prison in Siberia. There he experienced his first epileptic seizure. Dostoevsky's own epilepsy was particularly acute as he was writing the novel.

The Pickwick Papers
By Charles Dickens. IndyPublish.com pb, 2003, $18.99. (Originally published in 1837.) Fiction.
Among the most memorable of the many comic characters Dickens introduces in *The Pickwick Papers* is Joe, the narcoleptic servant of Mr. Tupman. According to the *DSM-IV*, narcolepsy—particularly in the extreme form exhibited by Joe—is rare; it would have occurred in as few as 3,600 of the approximately 18 million people in England and Wales at the midpoint of the 19th century.

4. The Inner Lives of Disordered Brains

By Anne Harrington, Ph.D.

From *Cerebrum: The Dana Forum on Brain Science,* Vol. 7, No. 2, Spring 2005 © Dana Press.

Aphasia and Kindred Disorders of Speech

By Sir Henry Head. Now available as The Classics of Neurology & Neurosurgery, Special edition, 1987. (Originally published in 1926.) $100.00. Non-fiction.

Includes an extensive case history of a young staff officer injured in World War I. A milestone in writing about patients with neurological trauma because it captured a change in social attitudes toward neurological patients. World War I had the effect of changing the typical neurological patient profile, which in turn brought the doctor-patient relationship onto more intimate and egalitarian lines.

Imaginary Portraits

By Walter Pater. IndyPublish.com, 2002, $22.99. (Originally published in 1887.) Fiction.

Rich interior descriptions of fictional characters, who functioned in part as psychological allegories. A favorite of teachers and students of literature, art history, and aesthetics.

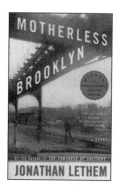
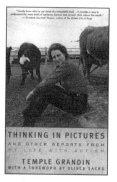
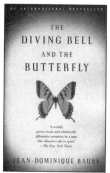
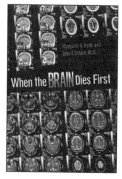

Motherless Brooklyn

By Jonathan Lethem. Vintage pb, 2000, $13.95. (Originally published in hardcover by Doubleday, 1999.) Fiction.

Told in the voice of a character with Tourette syndrome. Set in modern-day Brooklyn, Lionel Essrog works to uncover who murdered his boss and learns that his tics actually make him a better detective.

Partial View: An Alzheimer's Journal

By Cary Henderson. Southern Methodist University Press pb, 1998, $24.95. Non-fiction.

Describes the process of Alzheimer's from the inside, what it feels like little by little to lose one's memory and everyday moorings. Henderson recorded his increasingly disjointed thoughts onto a tape that was then edited by family members.

Phantoms in the Brain: Probing the Mysteries of the Human Mind

By V.S. Ramachandran. HarperPerennial pb, 1999, $16.00. (Originally published in hardcover by William Morris, 1998.) Non-fiction.

A description of the personal subjective experiences of Ramachandran's patients. He posits insights into mysterious conditions like anosognosia, phantom limb pain, and blindsight.

The Diving Bell and the Butterfly

By Jean-Dominique Bauby. Vintage pb, 1998, $11.95. (Originally published in hardcover by Knopf, 1997.) Non-fiction.

Describes what it's like to have one's intact subjectivity suddenly locked inside a body that will no longer move and can no longer speak. Bauby had an ultimately fatal stroke that resulted in a rare condition called "locked-in syndrome," leaving him able to move only his left eyelid.

The Man Who Tasted Shapes

By Richard Cytowic. MIT Press pb, 2003, $21.95. (Originally published in hardcover by G.P. Putnam's Sons, 1993.) Non-fiction.

An account of what it's like to live with synesthesia, a condition, according to the author, characterized by the prioritization of emotional knowledge over reason.

The Man With a Shattered World

By A.R. Luria. Harvard University Press, 2004, $17.95. (Originally published in hardcover by Basic Books, 1972). Non-fiction.

The story of a soldier, Zasetsky, who suffers brain damage and begins writing a journal to help put his thoughts, memories, and life back together. Told as a narrative in two voices, that of the patient as it comes through in excerpts from his journal, and that of his doctor, Luria himself, commenting on the patient's experiences and providing analytic context for making sense of them.

The Mind of a Mnemonist

By A.R. Luria. Harvard University Press pb, 2006, $18.95. (Originally published in hardcover by Basic Books, 1968.) Non-fiction.

A 30-year case history of a man who never forgot anything he experienced. This study of a man named Sherashevsky is Luria's "romantic" portrait of a "lost soul" whose indiscriminate memory made him unable to connect to the world.

Thinking in Pictures, Expanded Edition: My Life With Autism

By Temple Grandin. Vintage pb, 2006, $12.95. (Originally published in hardcover by Doubleday, 1995.) Non-fiction.

A woman with high-functioning autism points to ways which her highly visual, rational, and concrete form of thinking enables her to do things—such as designing more humane mechanisms for handling livestock—that so-called normal people cannot.

5. Four Fictional Odysseys Through Life With a Disordered Brain

By Todd E. Feinberg, M.D.

From *Cerebrum: The Dana Forum on Brain Science*, Vol. 7, No. 4, Fall 2005 © 2005 Dana Press.

Born Twice: A Novel of Fatherhood

By Giuseppe Pontiggia. Vintage pb, 2003, $13.00. (Originally published in hardcover by Knopf, 2002.) Fiction.

The story of how the members of a small family deal with each other, themselves, and the outside world in the face of their youngest child Paolo's

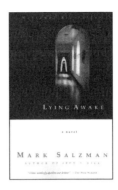
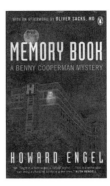

cerebral palsy. Narrated by the father, the aptly named Frigerio, whose greatest concern seems to be how to love his son, how to be a good, loving and caring father despite his true feelings about Paolo's difficulties.

Lying Awake

By Mark Salzman. Vintage pb, 2001, $12.00. (Originally published in hardcover by Knopf, 2000.) Fiction.

Sister John of the Cross has a religious epiphany for the first time in her life. At age 40, she has spent 20 years serving God dutifully in a monastery in the heart of Los Angeles, and now, finally, she feels fulfilled. Unfortunately, the seizures which caused the religious experience now threaten her health and Sister John's fellow nuns insist that she seek a neurological consultation.

Memory Book: A Benny Cooperman Mystery

By Howard Engel. Carroll & Graf pb, 2005, $13.95. (Originally published by Penguin Canada, 2005.) Fiction.

The victim of an attempted murder, private eye Benny Cooperman is found in a dumpster beside a dead woman. Having sustained massive head injuries and unable to remember the past, make new memories, or even read his own handwriting, Benny has to solve a mystery and clear his name from his bed in a Toronto rehabilitation facility.

The Speed of Dark

By Elizabeth Moon. Ballantine Books pb, 2004. $13.95. (Originally published in hardcover by Ballantine Books, 2003.) Fiction.

In a future America where science has all but eradicated autism, a stigma persists against those with even traces of the condition. Lou Arrendale's mild autism makes him a genius at his job doing pattern analysis for a large pharmaceutical company but renders him otherwise socially paralyzed. When a new genetic procedure that promises to reverse his autism becomes available, Lou has to decide if the change is worth it.

6. Brain Books for Budding Scientists—and All Children

By Carolyn Phelan
From *Cerebrum: The Dana Forum on Brain Science,* Vol. 4, No. 2, Summer 2002 © Dana Press.

101 Questions Your Brain Has Asked About Itself But Couldn't Answer...Until Now

By Faith Hickman Brynie. Millbrook Press, 1998, $25.90. Non-fiction.
Students' questions about the brain, paired with Brynie's answers, appear in seven chapters covering basic information, neurons, learning and memory, chemicals and drugs in the brain, damage and illness, left- and right-brain functions, and speech and the senses. Each chapter includes a related feature article on a topic such as brain imaging.

Head and Brain Injuries

By Elaine Landau. Enslow Publishers, 2002, $26.60. Non-fiction.
Landau surveys the most common forms of traumatic brain injuries, their causes and treatments, and how they change lives. In addition, she offers a brief historical survey of brain science and medical treatment.

Phineas Gage: A Gruesome but True Story About Brain Science

By John Fleischman. Houghton Mifflin pb, 2002, $16.00. (Originally published in hardcover by Houghton Mifflin, 2002.) Non-fiction.
Here is the story of the 19th-century railway worker who accidentally drove an iron tamping rod into his skull. This case study marked the beginning of a fuller understanding of the brain. Readers new to Gage's tale will come away intrigued by the story, knowledgeable about the brain, and (even better) curious to find out more.

When the Brain Dies First

By Margaret O. Hyde and John F. Setaro. Franklin Watts, 2000, $24.00. Non-fiction.
The authors begin with a brief introduction to the healthy brain, then zero in on the many things that can go wrong. They discuss injuries to the head; encephalitis and Creutzfeldt-Jakob disease; dementia caused by Alzheimer's disease; and degenerative diseases such as multiple sclerosis, among many other topics.

The Curious Incident of the Dog in the Night-Time

By Mark Haddon. Vintage pb, 2004, $12.95. (Originally published in hardcover by Doubleday, 2003.) Fiction.
Haddon, who once worked with autistic children and currently teaches creative writing, leads readers into the chaos of autism. He creates a character of such empathy that many readers will feel for the first time what it is like to live with no filters to eliminate or order the millions of pieces of information that stimulate our senses every moment. The protagonist, an autistic teen, investigates the murder of a neighbor's dog, entering and coping with an overwhelming outside world.

Chapter 7

Tracing Shakespeare's Insights Through Modern Brain Science

By Paul M. Matthews, M.D., and Jeffrey McQuain, Ph.D.

(Excerpted from *The Bard on the Brain: Understanding the Mind Through the Art of Shakespeare and the Science of Brain Imaging*, by Paul M. Matthews, M.D., and Jeffrey McQuain, Ph.D. Dana Press, Washington, DC, 2003. Reprinted with permission.)

From the Introduction:

For the people of England, the Elizabethan period was a time of enormous expansion in many spheres of life. The broadening of intellectual horizons throughout Europe established the foundations for the period of Enlightenment in the eighteenth century. It was a time of great economic and social change, during which England became a dominant European power. A key to this power was control of the seaways, by which explorations of the outside world proceeded ever more rapidly. And as new lands were being discovered, the nature of the European world was being redefined and the sense of human potential enlarged.

William Shakespeare both led and reflected his age. He developed the English language to an extent that no single writer has since. He mined the language of the rich and poor, rulers and the ruled, to develop more precise ways of expressing his thoughts and feelings. In doing so, he explored the inner world of man in a way that paralleled the journeys of the seafarers whose tales filled the taverns of England's ports....

What we appreciate as Shakespeare's genius derives from his keen insight into the human mind and from his obvious excitement in using this insight to experiment in drama. While his experiments were not designed and executed as are those of modern brain scientists, the underlying goals had intriguing similarities. His laboratory was the theater, where he tested his words and refined them until

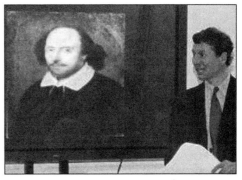

Paul M. Matthews, M.D., director of brain imaging at Oxford University, says that William Shakespeare provided exceptional insights on the brain and the mind in his characters. Modern brain researchers just now have the imaging tools to prove these observations.

they communicated powerfully and accurately. Like a modern brain scientist, he was testing hypotheses concerning the ways in which the human mind works. By using—and at the same time working to define—this complexity in his poetry and plays, he achieved his great art. In creating his enduring theater, Shakespeare also defines for us the uniqueness and wonder of the human mind....

In attempting to understand the mind, brain scientists finally have the means to address questions that Shakespeare so eloquently put forward four centuries ago.

Minds and Brains
(Seeing the Man Through His Brain)
Extract from Hamlet, *Act V, Sc. 1*

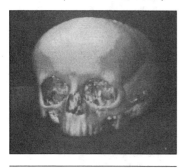

Self-reflection: Hamlet reveals the sensitivity of the brain to its own condition. (Daniel Travis, actor.)

The Shakespeare Theatre in Washington, DC, joined Dr. Paul Matthews in bringing selections from *The Bard on the Brain* to life. Students in drama and biology can increase their knowledge of the brain by doing the same.

Grasping the skull of a long-dead friend, Hamlet speaks what is perhaps the most misquoted line ever penned by Shakespeare: "Alas, poor Yorick, I knew him, Horatio" (not "I knew him well," as is so popularly believed). The Prince of Denmark's words come during a brief comic scene near the end of the play, when Hamlet meets a garrulous gravedigger. Hamlet does not yet know that his beloved Ophelia has drowned herself or that her grave is being prepared. When the gravedigger produces the skull of Yorick, once a jester to Hamlet's father, Hamlet fondly recalls the jester from his youth, now perhaps two decades past. Presaging the tragic news of Ophelia that is to follow, the skull reminds Hamlet that all of us must eventually die. Hamlet sees his former friend through his skull—a solid shell that can remain even after the brain is long decayed.

Hamlet: Alas, poor Yorick. I knew him, Horatio, a fellow of infinite jest, of most excellent fancy. He hath bore me on his back a thousand times, and now—how abhorred in my imagination it is. My gorge rises at it. Here hung those lips that I have kissed I know not how oft. Where be your gibes now, your gambols, your songs, your flashes of merriment, that were wont to set the table on a roar? Not one now to mock your own grinning? Quite chop-fallen? Now get you to my lady's chamber and tell her, let her paint an inch thick, to this favour she must come. Make her laugh at that.

Hamlet, 5.1

...Yorick's "most excellent fancy" must, of course, have arisen from the physical substance of his brain. A recurring theme in brain science (which also may have contributed to Shakespeare's beliefs concerning the brain) has been that the structure of the brain reflects its function in a rather direct way. People have even thought that the shape of the brain (which would be reflected in the shape of the inner surface of Yorick's skull) reflects an individual's personality, intellectual capacity, and moral character....

We do not now believe that character traits or brain functions can be localized in a simple way. Instead, it is felt that the brain processes information by means of complex networks of interactions between widely distributed regions of the brain—rather than solely in specific areas that might be reflected in local skull shape. Yet it is also clear that over the course of its development, the brain becomes regionally specialized for different functions. Perhaps one of the clearest examples of this is the way that regions specialized for processing language are highly lateralized to the left side of the brain in most people.

Language and Numbers
(A Subtle Voice)
Extract from* The Merchant of Venice, *Act IV, Sc. 1

Word choice is key to the poet's art. Novel words or turns of phrase are so striking to us that their novelty must influence the way in which the brain processes language. In The Merchant of Venice, *Portia speaks one of Shakespeare's most emotionally charged passages, which includes unexpected and novel word images. Dressed as a man, Portia enters a Venetian courtroom and passes herself off as Balthazar, a young doctor of laws from Rome. In the passage chosen here, Portia eloquently reminds the court of the "quality of mercy" that "droppeth" like rain and urges Shylock to be merciful toward the merchant Antonio. It is important to know that although Shylock remains unmoved by her impassioned arguments and demands that Antonio forfeit the promised pound of flesh, Portia's subtle voice eventually works its power and turns the tables on Shylock.*

Portia: The quality of mercy is not strain'd,
    It droppeth as the gentle rain from heaven
    Upon the place beneath: it is twice blest.
    It blesseth him that gives and him that takes,
    'Tis mightiest in the mightiest, it becomes
    The throned monarch better than his crown.
    His sceptre shows the force of temporal power,
    The attribute to awe and majesty,
    Wherein doth sit the dread and fear of kings:
    But mercy is above this sceptred sway,
    It is enthroned in the hearts of kings,
    It is an attribute to God himself;
    An earthly power doth then show likest God's
    When mercy seasons justice: Therefore Jew,
    Though justice be thy plea, consider this,
    That in the course of justice, none of us
    Should see salvation: we do pray for mercy,
    And that same prayer, doth teach us all to render
    The deeds of mercy. I have spoke thus much
    To mitigate the justice of thy plea,
    Which if thou follow, this strict court of Venice
    Must needs give sentence 'gainst the merchant there.
The Merchant of Venice, 4.1

One aspect of great poetry such as that of Shakespeare is the way in which the words resonate in our minds. As we read, "The quality of mercy is not strain'd/It droppeth as the gentle rain from heaven/Upon the place beneath," the words arrest our attention because of the beauty and uniqueness of both the metaphor and the sound. Why is it that the novelty of Shakespeare's words and their combinations adds so much to his poetry?

We respond to novelty in different ways than we respond to the over-familiar, and this is as true for words as it is for other inputs to the brain....[B]rain scientists [have] used the sensitive technique of magnetoencephalography (MEG) to study the patterns and relative timing of activations in the brain during a task that involved making a simple decision....[T]he MEG method detects the very tiny changes in magnetic fields produced by electrical activity in neurons.

Drugs and the Brain
(A Celebration of Alcohol)
Extract from **Henry IV, *Part II, Act IV, Sc. 3***

In various ways, Shakespeare both censures and celebrates the effects of alcohol on the human brain and body. For its celebration, he speaks through Falstaff, one of his most memorable characters and a man resolutely committed to drinking. In Henry IV, Part II, *Falstaff recounts the benefits of alcohol. Left alone onstage by the sober Prince John, Falstaff comically considers that some wine would help mellow the too-serious prince. As this prose monologue continues, he singles out Prince Henry (or Harry), John's older brother and the heir to the throne, as an example of one who has improved as a result of the effects of alcohol (a popular form of which at the time was "sherris-sack," a type of fortified wine similar to modern sherry).*

Falstaff: Good faith, this same young sober-blooded boy doth not love me, nor a man cannot make him laugh; but that's no marvel, he drinks no wine. There's never none of these demure boys come to any proof; for thin drink doth so over-cool their blood, and making many fish meals, that they fall into a kind of male green-sickness; and then when they marry they get wenches. They are generally fools and cowards—which some of us should be too, but for inflammation. A good sherris-sack hath a twofold operation in it. It ascends me into the brain, dries me there all the foolish and dull and crudy vapours which environ it, makes it apprehensive, quick, forgetive, full of nimble, fiery, and delectable shapes, which delivered o'er to the voice, the tongue, which is the birth, becomes excellent wit. The second property of your excellent sherris is the warming of the blood, which before, cold and settled, left the liver white and pale, which is the badge of pusillanimity and cowardice; but the sherris warms it and makes it course from the inwards to the parts, extremes. It illumineth the face, which, as a beacon, gives warning to all the rest of this little kingdom, man, to arm; and then the vital commoners, and inland petty spirits, muster me all to their captain, the heart; who, great and puffed up with this retinue, doth any deed of courage; and this valour comes of sherris. So that skill in the weapon is nothing without sack, for that sets it a-work, and learning a mere hoard of gold kept by a devil, till sack commences it and sets it in act and use. Hereof comes it that Prince Harry is valiant; for the cold blood he did naturally inherit of his father he hath like lean, sterile, and bare land manured, husbanded, and tilled, with excellent endeavour of drinking good and good store of fertile sherris, that he is become very hot and valiant. If I had a thousand sons, the first human principle I would teach them should be to forswear thin potations, and to addict themselves to sack.

Henry IV, Part II, 4.3

Falstaff is a rogue, a drunkard, and a coward. He is also the comic "life of the party" and deeply fond of his companions-in-carousing. But despite his rich good humor, one sees in him the tragic self-awareness of a life unfulfilled. His melancholy stems in part from recollections of slights, failures, and unmet expectations.

Falstaff has become enamored of the personality that he has generated for himself with the help of alcohol. His celebration of alcohol springs from the way it relieves self-doubt and banishes unpleasant memories. He needs to be freed from inhibitions arising from his own sense of unworthiness in order to enjoy himself. His celebration of alcohol is also interesting from a medical point of view because it both describes much that is true about this most common of drugs and includes myths that only a person "under the influence" (such as Falstaff) could propagate.

In trying to rationalize Prince John's dull seriousness, Falstaff concludes that part of the problem is that John simply "drinks no wine." Falstaff describes the effects of alcohol in reducing inhibition, claiming that "It ascends me into the brain, [and] dries me there all foolish and dull and crudy vapours," allowing his "excellent wit" to surface.

Alcohol of course has more general effects on the body. The "warming of the blood" that Falstaff refers to is not real but a feeling that comes from increased circulation due to alcohol-induced dilation of the small vessels of the skin. In consequence, it "illumineth the face, which, as a beacon, gives warning to all the rest of this little kingdom, man…"—the "warning" likely being simply that the drinker has had too much!

Falstaff describes alcohol from the standpoint of an unrepentant abuser of the drug. In fact, alcohol is a depressant of the nervous system. It makes speech appear "nimble" because it depresses brain functions responsible for self-monitoring and other processes that demand focused attention. This loss of effective self-monitoring underlies the partygoer's insistence that he can drive home safely, when everyone else can see that he is too drunk even to walk straight.

Decision and Action
(Motivation and Morality)
Extract from **Richard III,** *Act I, Sc. 1*

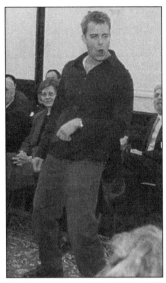

Sociopathic behavior: Richard III, in his own words, is "subtle, false, and treacherous" and lacks any sense of right or wrong. (Daniel Travis, actor.)

What motivates us to act (or not to act) is a central concern of Shakespeare's drama. Among the earliest of Shakespeare's history plays, Richard III *is also the only one of his plays to begin with a soliloquy by its title character. As the Duke of Gloucester and brother to King Edward IV, Richard makes his motivation all too clear in this introductory speech. Punning on "sun" and "son" in the opening sentence, he goes on to boast of his immoral scheme to usurp the crown, excusing his evil intentions with his physical deformity. He has set his plan in motion by promoting a prophecy that someone with the initial G will murder Edward's heirs. As a result, the king orders the arrest of George, the Duke of Clarence, brother to both the king and Richard, and unwittingly aids his evil brother's rise to become Richard III.*

Richard III: Now is the winter of our discontent
     Made glorious summer by this son of York;
     And all the clouds that lour'd upon our House
     In the deep bosom of the ocean buried.
     Now are our brows bound with victorious wreaths,
     Our bruised arms hung up for monuments,
     Our stern alarums chang'd to merry meetings,
     Our dreadful marches to delightful measures.
     Grim-visag'd War hath smooth'd his wrinkled front:
     And now, instead of mounting barded steeds
     To fright the souls of fearful adversaries,
     He capers nimbly in a lady's chamber,
     To the lascivious pleasing of a lute.
     But I, that am not shap'd for sportive tricks
     Nor made to court an amorous looking-glass;
     I, that am rudely stamp'd, and want love's majesty
     To strut before a wanton ambling nymph:
     I, that am curtail'd of this fair proportion,
     Cheated of feature by dissembling Nature,
     Deform'd, unfinish'd, sent before my time
     Into this breathing world scarce half made up—
     And that so lamely and unfashionable
     That dogs bark at me, as I halt by them—
     Why, I, in this weak piping time of peace,
     Have no delight to pass away the time,
     Unless to spy my shadow in the sun,
     And descant on mine own deformity.
     And therefore, since I cannot prove a lover
     To entertain these fair well-spoken days,
     I am determined to prove a villain,

And hate the idle pleasures of these days.
Plots have I laid, inductions dangerous,
By drunken prophecies, libels, and dreams,
To set my brother Clarence and the King
In deadly hate, the one against the other:
And if King Edward be as true and just
As I am subtle, false, and treacherous,
This day should Clarence closely be mew'd up
About a prophecy, which says that 'G'
Of Edward's heirs the murderer shall be—
Dive, thoughts, down to my soul: here Clarence
comes.

Richard III, 1.1

Richard III is particularly chilling as he describes his joint deformities of body and mind: "I, that am curtail'd of this fair proportion,/Cheated of feature by dissembling Nature,...I am determined to prove a villain." The horror of this passage is that a man could be so evil as to desire to harm others without specific cause. There is no motivation for revenge or power behind Richard's plan—he believes that he is "subtle, false, and treacherous" because to be so is quite simply in his nature.

Understanding the basis of moral action has been a challenge for Western literature since its beginnings in the great epics of the *Iliad* and the *Odyssey*. It is now becoming an important issue for modern brain science. We cannot help being fascinated by the enigma of Richard, who so clearly understands our moral universe and yet rejects its tenets. There is still no science that can explain the evil of Shakespeare's Richard, but brain scientists are beginning to define structures in the brain that are essential for aspects of moral and responsible behavior.

A critical aspect of moral behavior is the ability to forgo smaller, short-term gains in order to realize more distant but greater rewards. For example, a student learns to forgo the pleasures of a night out before examinations in order to achieve higher marks and the praise and new opportunities that arise from them. Patients who have suffered severe damage to the middle part of the frontal lobe such as Phineas Gage...have a childlike impulsiveness that prevents them from acting "responsibly" in this way. Nonetheless, patients who damage their brains as adults, like Gage, are at least able to appreciate the concepts behind this strategy.

Recent studies by Hannah and Antonio Damasio and their group at the University of Iowa suggest that this may not be the case if damage to the same areas of the brain occurs early in development. They studied two young adults who had sustained damage to the front part of the brain (the orbitofrontal and medial frontal cortices) before 16 months of age. ...Both had a history of severe family and social problems arising from irresponsibility, an inability to follow orders, and lack of guilt or remorse for misdeeds. However, not only were these subjects impaired in their moral behavior, like those who suffer similar lesions as adults, but they also showed defects in their ability to perform social and moral reasoning in the abstract. With early damage to this area of the brain, they simply were unable to appreciate the rules. These cases were clearly different from that of Phineas Gage...who retained an ability to distinguish between right and wrong.

Our Inner World
(Music as a Call to Life)
Extract from **The Winter's Tale,** *Act V, Sc. 3*

Music seems to have a magic all its own. Shakespeare recognizes this magic and dramatizes its potency in one of his later plays, The Winter's Tale. *Dramatic intensity is focused on the final scene of the play, in which music appears to bring a statue to life. At the beginning of the play, after the Sicilian king Leontes' jealous rage against her, his innocent wife, Hermione, wrongfully imprisoned for adultery, conspires to be reported dead. With this following the death of his only son, the lonely king repents his anger. Paulina, a faithful attendant of Hermione, then unveils a "statue" that proves to be a remarkably exact replica of the supposedly dead queen. In the scene that follows, after Paulina reawakens Leontes' faith in his wife, her demand for music acts as a seemingly magical call to life for the "statue."*

Paulina: Music, awake her; strike!

   [Music.]

   'Tis time; descend; be stone no more; approach;
   Strike all that look upon with marvel. Come!
   I'll fill your grave up: stir, nay, come away:
   Bequeath to death your numbness; for from him
   Dear life redeems you. You perceive she stirs:

   [Hermione comes down.]

   Start not; her actions shall be holy as
   You hear my spell is lawful.

   [to Leontes] Do not shun her
   Until you see her die again; for then
   You kill her double. Nay, present your hand:
   When she was young you woo'd her; now, in age,
   Is she become the suitor?

Leontes: O, she's warm!
   If this be magic, let it be an art
   Lawful as eating.

   The Winter's Tale, 5.3

The image of music calling a statue to life is striking. Who among us has not felt the compulsion to tap, rock, or gyrate wildly to the stimulating beat of a popular band? Music can animate the emotions as well as the body. Just as a stern face can melt into a smile on hearing a lively tune, so Hermione's apparently stony form dissolves into soft flesh with the sound of the music. Even without words, music communicates directly in ways that Shakespeare often used.

Shakespeare's plays are full of music, and he very consciously employs its power to move his audience. Songs such as the one at the end of *Twelfth Night*— "When that I was and a little tiny boy/With hey, ho, the wind and the rain,/ A foolish thing was but a toy,/For the rain it raineth every day"—provide an appropriate denouement, or rounding out of the action, at the close of an act. There also is often a real sense of music in the rhythm of Shakespeare's words and the timbre of their sounds.

Modern neuroscientists now appreciate that musical processing activates many parts of the brain. Research is being conducted in several laboratories to define precisely how music is perceived in the brain. Richard Frackowiak and his colleagues at the Functional Imaging Laboratory of University College in London are among those who performed some of the first neuroimaging studies of the effects of music on the brain. In their experiments using PET, they varied specific qualities of music for a group of listeners. By recording brain activity while changing pitch and rhythm independently, for example [they generated images which demonstrate that] processing of these specific musical elements is performed by large groups of nerve cells primarily found in the left side of the brain. There appears to be considerable overlap with areas of the brain that are used for language. For example, both language and rhythm activate the so-called superior temporal gyrus, the fold on the top of the lower lobe of the brain, and Broca's area, in the lower part of the front of the brain. This should probably not be surprising, as making sense of the sounds of words also must involve an appreciation of rhythm and pitch. One of the greatest difficulties with learning a foreign language, for instance, is appreciating the typical patterns of sounds that define words and sentences in that language.

In their studies of music, Frackowiak and his colleagues were surprised to find that variation of pitch discrimination primarily activated areas in the back of the brain that had previously been thought to be used primarily for visual perception. One possible explanation for this is that pitch decoding may involve a visual component. Mental imagery may be used in some way to encode patterns of relative pitch in music. If this is true, then when we speak colloquially of a musical pitch as being "higher" or "lower," it may be a reflection of a bias in the human brain for processing relationships in spatial terms.

Frackowiak's experiments also identified brain activity in the back part of the right side during judgments of timbre. This area (known as the right parietal lobe) is activated also (although obviously not exclusively) for tasks that demand thinking about spatial relations. Timbre may in some respects require a type of thinking analogous to spatial processing, because it involves understanding the relationships between different pure tones that make up the sound as a whole.

Together these observations illustrate how much of the brain is involved in the processing of music—suggesting how completely it can dominate our consciousness. Music truly calls the brain as a whole to life!

The Bard on the Brain:
Understanding the Mind Through the Art of Shakespeare and the Science of Brain Imaging

Table of Contents

A Note on Sources of Information on the Brain

The Dana Foundation provides many resources and offers directions to other sources to keep you informed of news on the cutting edge of brain research.

An Internet Connection for News on the Brain and Brain Research

www.dana.org serves as a gateway to the latest news and information on the brain and brain 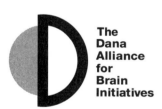 research. At the Brain Center you will learn more about the Dana Alliance for Brain Initiatives, a leading organization of pre-eminent neuroscientists dedicated to advancing public education about the brain in an understandable and accessible fashion. (For a complete listing of Dana Alliance members, please view the annual *Dana Alliance Progress Report on Brain Research* at www.dana.org.)

Brain Awareness Week^sm is an international effort organized by the Dana Alliance to advance public awareness about the progress and promise of brain research. Discover the activities planned in your locality and get involved in this educational campaign.

The Dana BrainWeb provides general information about the brain and current brain research, and links to validated sites related to more than 25 brain disorders. Brainy Kids Online offers children, parents, and teachers a site with activities for younger children, puzzles, links to excellent educational resources, and lesson plans. Brain Resources for Seniors provides older adults with links to sites related to brain health, education, and general information.

Brain Awareness Week^sm is a service mark of the Dana Alliance for Brain Initiatives.

Dana Press

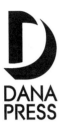

Dana Press, a division of the Dana Foundation, publishes health and popular science books about the brain for the general reader. It also publishes periodicals and educational material, as well as informational material on behalf of the Dana Foundation and Dana Alliance. (To subscribe to Dana Press free publications and periodicals, or to learn more about Dana Press books, visit www.dana.org/ books/press. Also, see specific publication information, below.)

Webcasts

Watch and listen to Webcasts from the Dana Centre in London, the Dana Center in Washington, DC, and other sites. The Webcasts focus on timely subjects, including brain research and neuroethics.

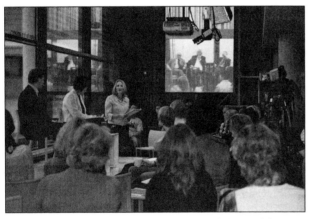

Dana Webcasts connect audiences around the world on current, science-related issues.

Podcasts

The Podcast section of www.dana.org features the latest in the Dana Alliance's award-winning *Gray Matters* radio series and other brain-related forums and discussions.

Radio and TV

Transcripts and audio are available for the award-winning *Gray Matters* radio series. Transcripts are available for the *Exploring Your Brain* television

series. Both are produced in association with the Dana Alliance.

Immunology and Arts Education

The Dana Foundation also supports research to learn how the body's immune system protects us against infections. The Foundation has extended its longtime interest in education to support innovative professional development programs leading to improved teaching of the performing arts in public schools. Learn more about the Dana Foundation's interests and programs in immunology and arts education at www.dana.org.

Other Dana Press Books and Periodicals

Books for General Readers (available in bookstores).

Hard Science, Hard Choices: Facts, Ethics, and Policies Guiding Brain Science Today

By Sandra J. Ackerman

Hard Science, Hard Choices presents a focused discussion of the leading questions prominent thinkers deal with in considering the facts, ethics, and policies guiding brain science today. Sandra Ackerman weaves their arguments and discussions into a concise narrative concentrating on the most significant and immediate ethical issues that have emerged from recent brain research in the areas of brain imaging, drugs and the brain, and new technology aimed at the brain. Paper, 200 pp. 1-1932594-02-7 $12.95

The Creating Brain: The Neuroscience of Genius

By Nancy C. Andreasen, M.D., Ph.D.

Andreasen, a renowned psychiatrist and best-selling author, explores how the brain achieves creative breakthroughs—in art, literature, science, and business—including such questions as how creative people are different and the difference between genius and intelligence. A unique appreciation of the arts that awe us together with an inspiring vision of how each of us can nurture and develop our creative capacity. (See excerpt, p. 27.) Cloth, 225 pp. 1-932594-07-8 $23.95

The Ethical Brain
By Michael S. Gazzaniga, Ph.D.
Explores how the lessons of neuroscience can help us resolve today's ethical dilemmas, ranging from when life begins to "off-label" use of drugs such as Ritalin by students preparing for exams, and from free will and personal responsibility to public policy and religious belief. The author, a pioneer in cognitive neuroscience, is a member of the President's Council on Bioethics. (See excerpt, p. 32.) Cloth, 225 pp. 1-932594-01-9 $25.00

Fatal Sequence: The Killer Within
By Kevin J. Tracey, M.D.
An easily understood account of the body's ability to go into the fatal spiral of sepsis, a crisis that most often affects patients fighting off nonfatal illness or injury. Tracey puts the scientific and medical story of sepsis in the context of his battle to save a burned baby, a sensitive telling that renders cutting-edge science human and unforgettable. Cloth, 225 pp. 1-932594-06-X $23.95. Paper, 225 pp. 1-932594-09-4 $12.95

A Well-Tempered Mind: Using Music to Help Children Listen and Learn
By Peter Perret and Janet Fox
Five musicians enter elementary school classrooms, helping children learn about music and contributing both to higher enthusiasm and improved academic performance. This charming story gives us a taste of things to come in one of the newest areas of brain research: the effect of music on the brain. (See excerpt, p. 29.)
Cloth, 12 illustrations, 225 pp. 1-932594-03-5 $22.95. Paper, 12 illustrations, 225 pp., 1-932594-08-6 $12.95

A Good Start in Life: Understanding Your Child's Brain and Behavior from Birth to Age 6
By Norbert Herschkowitz, M.D.,* and Elinore Chapman Herschkowitz
Updated with the latest information and new material, the authors show us how young children learn to live together in family and society and explain how brain development shapes a child's personality and behavior, discussing appropriate rule-setting, the child's moral sense, temperament, language, playing, aggression, impulse control, and empathy. (See excerpt, p. 38.) Cloth, 283 pp. 0-309-07639-0 $22.95. (Updated version with 13 illustrations)
Paper, 312 pp. 0-9723830-5-0 $13.95
*Member of the European Dana Alliance for the Brain.

Neuroscience and the Law: Brain, Mind, and the Scales of Justice
Brent Garland, Editor. Foreword by Mark S. Frankel. With commissioned papers by Michael S. Gazzaniga, Ph.D., and Megan S. Steven; Laurence R. Tancredi, M.D., J.D.; Henry T. Greely, J.D.; and Stephen J. Morse, J.D., Ph.D.
How discoveries in neuroscience influence criminal and civil justice, based on an invitational meeting of 26 top neuroscientists, legal scholars, attorneys, and state and federal judges convened by the Dana Foundation and the American Association for the Advancement of Science. Paper, 226 pp. 1-932594-04-3 $8.95

Beyond Therapy: Biotechnology and the Pursuit of Happiness.
A Report of the President's Council on Bioethics
Special Foreword by Leon R. Kass, M.D., Chairman. Introduction by William Safire
Can biotechnology satisfy deep and familiar human desires—for better children, superior performance, ageless bodies, and happy souls? This landmark report says these possibilities present us with profound ethical challenges and choices. Paper, 376 pp. 1-932594-05-1 $10.95

Neuroethics: Mapping the Field.

Conference Proceedings

Steven J. Marcus, Editor

Proceedings of the landmark 2002 conference organized by Stanford University and the University of California, San Francisco, at which more than 150 neuroscientists, bioethicists, psychiatrists and psychologists, philosophers, and professors of law and public policy debated the implications of neuroscience research findings for individual and societal decision-making. 50 illustrations, Paper, 367 pp. 0-9723830-0-X $10.95

Back From the Brink: How Crises Spur Doctors to New Discoveries About the Brain

By Edward J. Sylvester

Goes into two academic medical centers, Columbia's New York Presbyterian and Johns Hopkins Medical Institutions, to watch a new breed of doctor, the neurointensivist, save patients with life-threatening brain injuries. (See excerpt, p. 33.) 16 illustrations/photos, Cloth, 296 pp. 0-9723830-4-2 $25.00

The Bard on the Brain: Understanding the Mind Through the Art of Shakespeare and the Science of Brain Imaging

*By **Paul Matthews, M.D.**,* and Jeffrey McQuain, Ph.D. Foreword by Diane Ackerman*

Explores the beauty and mystery of the human mind and the workings of the brain, following the path the Bard pointed out in 35 of the most famous speeches from his plays. (See excerpt, p. 83.) 100 illustrations, Cloth, 248 pp. 0-9723830-2-6 $35.00

*Member of the European Dana Alliance for the Brain

Striking Back At Stroke: A Doctor-Patient Journal

*By Cleo Hutton and **Louis R. Caplan, M.D.***

A personal account with medical guidance for anyone enduring the changes that a stroke can bring to a life, a family, and a sense of self. 15 illustrations. (See excerpt, p. 35.) Cloth, 240 pp. 0-9723830-1-8 $27.00

The Dana Guide to Brain Health

*Floyd E. Bloom, M.D., M. Flint Beal, M.D., and David J. Kupfer, M.D., Editors. Foreword by **William Safire***

A home reference on the brain edited by three leading experts collaborating with 104 distinguished scientists and medical professionals. In easy-to-understand language with cross-references and advice on 72 conditions such as autism, Alzheimer's disease, multiple sclerosis, depression, and Parkinson's disease. (See excerpt, p. 34.) 16 full-color pages and more than 200 black-and-white illustrations, Cloth, 768 pp. 0-7432-0397-6 $45.00

Understanding Depression: What We Know and What You Can Do About It

*By **J. Raymond DePaulo, Jr., M.D.**, and Leslie Alan Horvitz. Foreword by **Kay Redfield Jamison, Ph.D.***

What depression is, who gets it and why, what happens in the brain, troubles that come with the illness, and the treatments that work. (See excerpt, p. 37.) Cloth, 304 pp. 0-471-39552-8 $24.95. Paper, 296 pp. 0-471-43030-7 $14.95

Keep Your Brain Young: The Complete Guide to Physical and Emotional Health and Longevity

*By **Guy M. McKhann, M.D.**, and **Marilyn Albert, Ph.D.***

Every aspect of aging and the brain: changes in memory, nutrition, mood, sleep, and sex, as well as the later problems in alcohol use, vision, hearing, movement, and balance. (See excerpt, p. 42.) Cloth, 304 pp. 0-471-40792-5 $24.95. Paper, 304 pp. 0-471-43028-5 $15.95

The End of Stress As We Know It

*By **Bruce S. McEwen, Ph.D.**, with Elizabeth N. Lasley. Foreword by Robert Sapolsky*

How brain and body work under stress and how it is possible to avoid its debilitating effects. (See excerpt, p. 40.) Cloth, 239 pp. 0-309-07640-4 $27.95. Paper, 262 pp. 0-309-09121-7 $19.95

In Search of the Lost Cord: Solving the Mystery of Spinal Cord Regeneration

By Luba Vikhanski

The story of the scientists and science involved in the international scientific race to find ways to repair the damaged spinal cord and restore movement. (See excerpt, p. 39.) 21 photos; 12 illustrations, Cloth, 269 pp. 0-309-07437-1 $27.95

The Secret Life of the Brain

*By **Richard M. Restak**, M.D. Foreword by David Grubin*

Companion book to the PBS series of the same name, exploring recent discoveries about the brain from infancy through old age. Cloth, 201 pp. 0-309-07435-5 $35.00

The Longevity Strategy: How to Live to 100 Using the Brain-Body Connection

*By **David Mahoney** and **Richard M. Restak**, M.D. Foreword by **William Safire***

Advice on the brain and aging well. (See excerpt, p. 45.) Cloth, 250 pp. 0-471-24867-3 $22.95. Paper, 272 pp. 0-471-32794-8 $14.95

States of Mind: New Discoveries About How Our Brains Make Us Who We Are

Roberta Conlan, Editor

Adapted from the Dana/Smithsonian Associates lecture series by eight of the country's top brain scientists, including the 2000 Nobel laureate in medicine, Eric R. Kandel, M.D. (See excerpt, p. 44.) Cloth, 214 pp. 0-471-29963-4 $24.95. Paper, 224 pp. 0-471-39973-6 $18.95

Free Educational Books (order through www.dana.org)

The Dana Sourcebook of Immunology: Resources for Secondary and Post-Secondary Teachers and Students

Dan Gordon, Editor

An introduction to how the immune system protects us, what happens when it breaks down, the diseases that threaten it, and the unique relationship between the immune system and the brain. 5 color photos; 35 black-and-white photos; 11 black-and-white illustrations, 116 pp.

Partnering Arts Education: A Working Model from ArtsConnection

This publication illustrates the importance of classroom teachers and artists learning to form partnerships as they build successful residencies in schools. *Partnering Arts Education* provides insight and concrete steps in the ArtsConnection model. 55 pp.

Acts of Achievement: The Role of Performing Arts Centers in Education

Profiles of 60-plus programs, eight extended case studies, from urban and rural communities across the United States, illustrating different approaches to performing arts education programs in school settings. Black-and-white photos throughout, 164 pp.

Planning an Arts-Centered School: A Handbook

A practical guide for those interested in creating, maintaining, or upgrading arts-centered schools. Includes curriculum and development, governance, funding, assessment, and community participation. Black-and-white photos throughout, 164 pp.

Periodicals

The Brain in the News

A monthly, eight-page newspaper reprinting news and feature articles about brain research from leading newspapers and magazines in the United States and abroad during the previous month.
Free: order through www.dana.org/books/press

Cerebrum: The Dana Forum on Brain Science

A free monthly online journal for general readers with feature articles, book reviews, and book excerpts dealing with the latest discoveries about the brain and their implications for individuals and society. Both current issues and a full, searchable archive of *Cerebrum* print edition articles, book reviews, and book excerpts (1998-2005) is available at www.dana.org/books/press.
For more information, e-mail cerebrum@dana.org.

BrainWork: The Neuroscience Newsletter

A bimonthly, full-color, eight-page newsletter for general readers reporting the latest findings in brain research.
Free: order through or download from www.dana.org/books/press

Immunology in the News

A quarterly, eight-page newspaper reprinting news and feature articles about immune system research, disease treatment and prevention, and biodefense from U.S. and foreign newspapers and scientific journals.
Free: order through www.dana.org/books/press

Progress Report on Brain Research

Published in March annually since 1995, the *Progress Report,* a publication of the Dana Alliance for Brain Initiatives, identifies the most significant findings in brain research from the previous year.
Free: order through or download from www.dana.org/books/press

Brain Connections: Your Source Guide to Information on Brain Diseases and Disorders

Pocket-size, 48-page booklet listing more than 240 organizations that help people with a brain-related disorder and those responsible for their care and treatment. A publication of the Dana Alliance for Brain Initiatives. Listings include toll-free numbers, Web site and e-mail addresses, and mailing addresses.
Free: order through or download from www.dana.org/books/press

Arts Education in the News

A bimonthly, eight-page newspaper reprinting news and feature articles about performing arts education in the schools from leading U.S. and foreign newspapers and magazines.
Free: order through www.dana.org/books/press

A Glossary of Key Brain Science Terms

(Italicized terms are defined within this glossary.)

adrenal glands: Located on top of each kidney, these two glands are involved in the body's response to stress and help regulate growth, blood *glucose* levels, and the body's *metabolic* rate. They receive signals from the brain and secrete several different *hormones* in response, including *cortisol* and *adrenaline*.

adrenaline: Also called epinephrine, this *hormone* is secreted by the *adrenal glands* in response to stress and other challenges to the body. The release of adrenaline causes a number of changes throughout the body, including the *metabolism* of carbohydrates, to supply the body's energy demands.

allele: One of the variant forms of a *gene* at a particular location on a chromosome. Differing alleles produce variation in inherited characteristics such as hair color or blood type. In an individual, one form of the allele (the *dominant* one) may be expressed if one copy is present, while a *recessive* allele will show only where both copies are present.

amino acid: One of a group of 20 different kinds of small molecules that contain nitrogen as well as carbon, hydrogen, and oxygen that link together in folded chains to form proteins. Often referred to as the "building blocks" of proteins.

amino acid neurotransmitters: The most prevalent *neurotransmitters* in the brain, these include glutamate and aspartate, which have excitatory actions, and glycine and gamma-amino butyric acid (GABA), which have inhibitory actions.

amygdala: Part of the brain's *limbic system,* this primitive brain structure lies deep in the center of the brain and is involved in emotional reactions such as anger, as well as emotionally charged *memories.* It also influences behavior such as feeding, sexual interest, and the immediate "fight or flight" reaction to stress, to help ensure that the body's needs are met.

amyloid-b (Ab) protein: A naturally occurring protein in brain cells. Tangles of this protein form the plaques that are the hallmark of Alzheimer's disease and are thought by many researchers to cause the disease itself.

animal model: A scientific technique that relies on laboratory animals (usually mice or rats) to mimic specific behavioral traits or symptoms of a human disease. Many of the most promising advances in treating brain disorders have come from research on animal models.

astrocyte: Cell that delivers "fuel" to the *neurons* from the blood, removes waste from the *neuron,* and modulates the activity of the *neuron.*

auditory cortex: Part of the brain's *temporal lobe* (see Figure 3, p. 112), this is the area of the brain responsible for hearing. Nerve fibers extending from the inner ear carry nerve impulses generated by sounds into the auditory cortex for interpretation.

autonomic nervous system: Part of the *central nervous system* that controls functions of internal organs (e.g., blood pressure, respiration, intestinal function, urinary bladder control, perspiration, body temperature). Its actions are mainly involuntary.

axon: A long, single nerve fiber that transmits messages, via chemical and electrical impulses, from the body of the *neuron* to *dendrites* of other *neurons,* or directly to body tissues such as muscles. (See Figure 4, p. 113)

basal ganglia: Structure below the cortex involved in motor, *cognitive,* and emotional functions.

brain imaging: Refers to various techniques, such as *magnetic resonance imaging (MRI)* and *positron emission tomography (PET),* that enable scientists to capture images of brain tissue and structure and to reveal what parts of the brain are associated with various behaviors or activities.

brain stem: A primitive part of the brain that connects the brain to the *spinal cord.* The brain stem controls functions basic to the survival of all animals, such as heart rate, breathing, digestive processes, and sleeping. (See Figure 1, p. 110)

central nervous system: The brain and *spinal cord* constitute the central nervous system and are part of the broader nervous system, which also includes the *peripheral nervous system.*

central sulcus: The primary groove in the brain's *cerebrum,* which separates the *frontal lobe* in the front of the brain from the *parietal* and *occipital lobes* in the rear of the brain. (See Figure 3, p. 112.)

cerebellum: A brain structure located at the top of the *brain stem* (see Figure 1, p. 110) that coordinates the brain's instructions for skilled, repetitive movements and helps maintain balance and posture. Recent research also suggests the cerebellum may play a role, along with the *cerebrum,* in higher *cognitive* processes.

cerebrum (also called cerebral cortex): The largest brain structure in humans, accounting for about two-thirds of the brain's mass and positioned over and around most other brain structures. (See Figure 2, p. 111.) The cerebrum is divided into left and right *hemispheres,* as well as specific areas called lobes that are associated with specialized functions.

cognition: A general term that includes thinking, perceiving, recognizing, conceiving, judging, sensing, reasoning, and imagining. Also, cognitive, an adjective pertaining to cognition, as in cognitive processes.

computed tomography (CT or CAT): An X-ray technique introduced in the early 1970s that enables scientists to take cross-sectional images of the body and brain. CT uses an X-ray beam passed through the body to collect information about tissue density, then applies sophisticated computer and mathematical formulas to create an anatomical image from that data.

consciousness: The state of being aware of one's feelings and what is happening around one; the totality of one's thoughts, feelings, and impressions about the world around us. The search for the basis of consciousness in the activity and structures of the brain is one of the most intriguing areas of modern *neuroscience.*

cortisol: A steroid *hormone* produced by the *adrenal glands* that controls how the body uses fat, protein, carbohydrates, and minerals and helps reduce inflammation. Cortisol is released in the body's stress response; brain scientists have found that prolonged exposure to cortisol has damaging effects on the brain.

CT scan (also called CAT scan): See *computed tomography.*

dementia: General mental deterioration from a previously normal state of *cognitive* function due to disease or psychological factors (not to be confused with mental retardation, or developmental disability). Alzheimer's disease is one form of dementia.

dendrites: Short nerve fibers that project from a nerve cell, generally receiving messages from the *axons* of other *neurons* and relaying them to the cell's nucleus. (See Figure 4, p. 113)

dependence: In reference to drug or alcohol addiction, dependence describes a state marked by uncontrolled, compulsive drug use, in which the brain's "pleasure pathways"—networks of *neurons* that use the *neurotransmitter dopamine*—physically change, leading to drug dependency. (Also see *psychological dependence.*)

depression: A mood or affective disorder often characterized by disruptions in one or more of the brain's *neurotransmitter* systems, including those related to *serotonin* and *dopamine*. Clinical depression is a serious condition that can be effectively treated with medications and/or behavioral therapy.

DNA (deoxyribonucleic acid): The material from which the 46 chromosomes in each cell's nucleus is formed. DNA contains the codes for the body's approximately 30,000 *genes,* governing all aspects of cell growth and inheritance. DNA has a *double-helix* structure—two intertwined strands resembling a spiraling ladder.

dominant: A *gene* that almost always results in a specific physical characteristic, for example a disease, even though the patient's *genome* possesses only one copy. With a dominant *gene,* the chance of passing on the *gene* (and therefore the trait or disease) to children is 50-50 in each pregnancy.

dopamine: A *neurotransmitter* involved in the brain's reward, or pleasure, system and in the control of body movement. Some addictive drugs increase brain levels of dopamine, causing the "high" associated with illicit drug use. Virtually all addictive substances, from nicotine to alcohol to heroin and crack cocaine, affect the dopamine system in one way or another.

double helix: The structural arrangement of *DNA,* which looks something like an immensely long ladder twisted into a helix, or coil. The sides of the "ladder" are formed by a backbone of sugar and phosphate molecules, and the "rungs" consist of nucleotide bases joined weakly in the middle by hydrogen bonds.

endocrine system: A body system composed of several different glands and organs that secrete *hormones.*

endorphins: *Hormones* produced by the brain in response to pain or stress to blunt the sensation of pain. *Narcotic* drugs such as morphine imitate the actions of the body's natural endorphins.

enzyme: A protein that encourages a biochemical reaction, usually speeding it up. Organisms could not function if they had no enzymes.

frontal lobe: The front part of the brain's *cerebrum,* beneath the forehead. (See Figure 3, p. 112.) This area of the brain is associated with higher *cognitive* processes, such as decision-making, reasoning, and planning.

functional magnetic resonance imaging (fMRI): A *brain imaging* technique based on conventional *MRI,* but which uses sophisticated computer programs to create images that show which areas of the brain are functioning during certain tasks, behaviors, or thoughts.

gene: The basic unit of inheritance. A distinct section of *DNA* in a cell's chromosome that contains the codes for producing specific proteins involved in brain and body function. Gene defects (genetic *mutations*) are thought to cause many brain disorders.

gene expression: The process by which proteins are made from the instructions encoded in *DNA*.

gene mapping: Determining the relative positions of *genes* on a chromosome and the distance between them.

genome: The complete genetic map for an organism. In humans, this includes about 30,000 *genes* whose codes are written in our *DNA*, the spiraling chain of proteins that makes up the 46 chromosomes in each cell. More than 15,000 *genes* relate to functions of the brain.

glial cells: The supporting cells of the *central nervous system*. Though probably not involved directly in the transmission of nerve signals, glial cells protect and nourish the *neurons*.

glucose: A natural sugar that is carried in the blood and is the principal source of energy for the cells of the brain and body. *PET* imaging techniques measure brain activity by measuring increases in the brain's *metabolism* of glucose during specific mental tasks a person performs.

gray matter: The parts of the brain and spinal cord made up primarily of groups of *neuron* cell bodies (as opposed to *white matter*, which is composed mainly of *myelinated* nerve fibers).

gyrus: The ridges on the brain's outer surface. Plural is *gyri*.

haplotype: The set of SNP *alleles* (see description and graphic, p. 21) along a region of a chromosome. Theoretically there could be many haplotypes in a chromosome region, but recent studies are typically finding only a few common haplotypes. Understanding genetic variation will be essential to understanding complex genetic diseases that affect the brain and nervous system.

hemisphere: In brain science, refers to the two halves of the brain (the left and right hemispheres), which are separated by a deep groove, or fissure, down the center. Some major, specific brain functions are located in one or the other hemisphere.

hippocampus: A primitive brain structure located deep in the brain (see Figure 2, p. 111) that is involved in *memory* and learning.

hormone: A chemical released by the body's *endocrine* glands (including the *adrenal glands*), as well as by some tissues. Hormones act on *receptors* in other parts of the body to influence body functions or behavior.

hypothalamus: A small structure located at the base of the brain, where signals from the brain and the body's *hormonal* system interact (see Figure 2, p. 111).

interneuronal: Between *neurons*, as in interneuronal communication.

ions: Atoms or groups of atoms carrying a negative or positive charge of electricity. When a nerve impulse is fired, ions flow through channels in the membrane of a nerve cell, changing the charge in that local area of the cell to positive from its resting, negatively charged state. This sets off a chain reaction of positive charges that carries the nerve impulse along the cell's *axon* to the *synapse*, where it releases *neurotransmitters* into the *synaptic cleft*. (See Figures 5 and 6, pp. 114, 115.)

lesion: An injury or surgical incision to body tissue. Much of what has been learned about the functions of various brain structures or pathways has resulted from lesion studies, in which scientists observe the behavior of persons who have suffered injury to a distinct area of the brain or analyze the behavior resulting from a lesion made in the brain of a laboratory animal.

limbic system: A term for a group of brain structures that has probably changed little throughout evolution and is located in the inner brain, encircling the top of the *brain stem.* The limbic structures play a complex role in emotions, instincts, and behavioral drives.

magnetic resonance imaging (MRI): A *brain imaging* technique that uses intensely powerful magnets (some as much as 80,000 times the magnetic field of the Earth) to create sharp anatomical images of the brain or body. During an MRI scan, the person is placed inside a scanner, where the strong magnetic field causes the millions of atoms in the body to line up in a particular fashion (just as the needle of a compass lines up with the Earth's magnetic field). The machine then sends out pulses of radio waves, which cause the atoms to release radio signals. The pattern of signals provides information about the number of particular atoms present and their chemical environment. Sophisticated computer programs are then used to reconstruct the data into images of anatomical structure. MRI is also used to measure brain activity. (See *functional MRI.*)

melatonin: A *hormone* that is secreted by the pineal gland in the brain in response to the daily light-dark cycle, influencing the body's sleep-wake cycle and possibly affecting sexual development.

memory: A complex brain function that involves integrated systems of *neurons* in diverse brain areas, each of which handles individual memory-related tasks. Memory can be categorized into two distinct types, each with its own corresponding brain areas. Memory about people, places, and things is referred to as explicit or declarative memory and seems to be centered in the *hippocampus* and *temporal lobe.* (See Figures 2 and 3, pp. 111, 112.) Memory about motor skills and perceptual strategies is known as implicit, or procedural memory and seems to involve the *cerebellum*, the *amygdala* (see Figures 2 and 3, pp. 111, 112.), and specific pathways related to the particular skill (e.g., riding a bicycle would involve the *motor cortex*, etc.).

metabolize: To break down or build up biochemical elements in the body, effecting a change in body tissue. Brain cells metabolize *glucose,* a blood sugar, to derive energy for transmitting nerve impulses.

molecular biology: The study of the structure and function of cells at the level of the molecules from which they are comprised and how these molecules influence behavior and disease processes. Molecular biology has emerged as a scientific discipline only in the last couple of decades, due to advances in genetics and sophisticated technologies that have made it possible to "split" cells and study their internal structures.

motor cortex: The part of the brain's *cerebrum,* just to the front of the *central sulcus* in the *frontal lobe* (see Figure 3, p. 112), that is involved in movement and muscle coordination. Scientists have identified specific spots in the motor cortex that control movement in specific parts of the body, the so-called "motor map."

MRI: See *magnetic resonance imaging* and/or *functional magnetic resonance imaging.*

mutation: A permanent structural alteration in *DNA.* In most cases, *DNA* changes either have no effect or cause harm, but occasionally a mutation can improve an organism's chance of surviving and passing the beneficial change on to its descendants.

myelin: The fatty substance that sheaths most nerve cell *axons,* helping to insulate and protect the nerve fiber and helping to speed up the transmission of nerve impulses. (See Figure 4, p. 113.)

narcotic: A synthetic chemical compound that mimics the action of the body's natural *endorphins, hormones* secreted to counteract pain. Narcotic drugs have a valid and useful role in the management of pain but may lead to physical *dependence* in susceptible individuals if used for long periods.

neurodegenerative diseases: Diseases characterized by progressive deterioration of nerve cells (neurodegeneration). Neurodegenerative diseases include amyotrophic lateral sclerosis (also known as Lou Gehrig's disease), Huntington's disease, Alzheimer's disease, and Parkinson's disease.

neuroethics: A new interdisciplinary field of study that has arisen to address the ethical issues of our increased ability to understand and change the brain. Privacy, life extension, fairness, cloning, and many other issues are included in this ongoing social-scientific debate.

neurogenesis: The birth of new *neurons,* suspected since the mid 1950s to occur in the adult brain, but conclusive evidence emerged only as recently as 1998. Recent studies found that new *neurons* are vital to learning and *memory* and may help protect the brain against stress and *depression.* Neural *stem cells,* undifferentiated *stem cells* that grow up into *neurons* and *glial cells,* offer hope of treating many brain disorders, particularly the *neurodegenerative diseases* that involve the death of key brain cells.

neuroimmunology: A complex field in biomedical research whose work focuses on the brain, the immune system, and their interactions. Neuroimmunology holds the potential for conquering ills as diverse as *spinal cord* injury, multiple sclerosis, and bodily reactions to pathogens, both naturally occurring and intentionally inflicted.

neuron: Nerve cell. The basic units of the *central nervous system*, neurons are responsible for the transmission of nerve impulses. (See Figures 4 and 5, pp. 113, 114.) Unlike any other cell in the body, neurons consist of a central cell body as well as several threadlike "arms" called *axons* and *dendrites*, which transmit nerve impulses. Scientists estimate there are more than 100 billion neurons in the brain.

neuroscience: The study of the brain and nervous systems, including their structure, function, and disorders. Neuroscience as a discipline has emerged only in the last couple of decades.

neurotransmitter: A chemical that acts as a messenger between *neurons* and is released into the *synaptic cleft* when a nerve impulse reaches the end of an *axon*. (See Figures 5 and 6, pp. 114, 115.) Several dozen neurotransmitters have been identified in the brain so far, each with specific, often complex roles in brain function and human behavior.

nurture: In science, refers to the influence of environmental factors, such as the experiences one is exposed to in early life, in human development. The term is often used in the context of "nature versus nurture," which relates to the interplay of "nature" (genetic or inherited, predetermined influences) and environmental, or experiential, forces.

occipital lobe: A part of the brain's *cerebrum*, located at the rear of the brain, above the *cerebellum*. (See Figure 3, p. 112.) The occipital lobe is primarily concerned with vision and encompasses the *visual cortex*.

olfactory: Pertaining to the sense of smell. When stimulated by an odor, olfactory *receptor* cells in the nose send nerve impulses to the brain's olfactory bulbs, which in turn transmit the impulses to olfactory centers in the brain for interpretation.

opiate: A naturally occurring chemical that has specific actions in the brain, influencing the "pleasure pathways" of the *dopamine* system by locking onto specialized opiate *receptors* in certain *neurons*.

pain receptors: Specialized nerve fibers in the skin and on the surfaces of internal organs, which detect painful stimuli and send signals to the brain.

parietal lobe: The area of the brain's *cerebrum* located just behind the *central sulcus*. (See Figure 3, p. 112.) It is concerned primarily with the reception and processing of sensory information from the body and is also involved in map interpretation and spatial orientation (recognizing one's position in space vis-a-vis other objects or places).

peripheral nervous system: The nervous system outside the brain and *spinal cord*.

PET: See *positron emission tomography.*

physical dependence: See *dependence.*

pituitary gland: An *endocrine* organ closely linked with the *hypothalamus*. The pituitary gland is composed of two lobes and secretes a number of *hormones* that regulate the activity of the other *endocrine* organs in the body.

plasticity: In *neuroscience,* refers to the brain's capacity to change and adapt in response to developmental forces, learning processes, or aging, or in response to an injury in a distinct area of the brain.

positron emission tomography (PET): A *brain imaging* technique that measures changes in brain *metabolism* to create three-dimensional images of brain activity. In a PET scan, a radioactive "marker" that emits, or releases, positrons (parts of an atom that release gamma radiation) is injected into the bloodstream. Detectors outside of the head can sense these "positron emissions," which are then reconstructed using sophisticated computer programs to create "tomographs," or computer images. Since blood flow and *metabolism* increase in brain regions at work, those areas have higher concentrations of the marker, and researchers are able to see which brain regions are activated during certain tasks or exposure to sensory stimuli.

postsynaptic cell: The *neuron* on the receiving end of a nerve impulse transmitted from another *neuron*. (See Figure 5, p. 138.)

prefrontal cortex: The area of the *cerebrum* located in the forward part of the *frontal lobe* (see Figure 3, p. 112), which is thought to control higher *cognitive* processes such as planning, reasoning, and "social cognition"—a complex skill involving the ability to assess social situations in light of previous experience and personal knowledge and interact appropriately with others. The prefrontal cortex is thought to be the most recently evolved area of the brain.

premotor cortex: The area of the *cerebrum* located between the *prefrontal cortex* and the *motor cortex*, in the *frontal lobe*. (See Figure 3, p. 112.) It is involved in the planning and execution of movements.

presynaptic cell: In *synaptic transmission,* the *neuron* that sends a nerve impulse across the *synaptic cleft* to another *neuron*. (See Figure 5, p. 114.)

psychiatry: A medical specialty dealing with the diagnosis and treatment of mental disorders. (Contrast with *psychology*.)

psychoactive drug: A class of pharmaceutical medications that acts on the brain's pleasure and mood-regulating systems and can help control the symptoms of some neurological and *psychiatric* disorders, such as schizophrenia or obsessive-compulsive disorder.

psychological dependence: In the science of addiction, refers to what was once considered the psychological or behavioral aspects of addiction (such as craving a cigarette after a meal). Brain scientists now understand that psychological factors are central to addictive disorders and are often the most difficult to treat. (Also see *dependence.*)

psychology: An academic or scientific field of study concerned with the behavior of humans and animals and related mental processes. (Contrast to *psychiatry.*)

quadrillion: A number represented by 1 with 15 zeros (1,000,000,000,000,000). Scientists estimate that there are about 1 quadrillion *synaptic* connections between the *neurons* in the *central nervous system,* an estimate based on the belief that there are at least 100 billion (100,000,000,000) *neurons,* and that each *neuron* makes as many as 10,000 connections.

receptors: Molecules on the surfaces of *neurons* whose structures precisely match those of chemical messengers (such as *neurotransmitters* or *hormones*) released during *synaptic transmission.* The chemicals attach themselves to the receptors, in lock-and-key fashion, to activate the receiving cell structure (usually a *dendrite* or cell body). (See Figures 5 and 6, pp. 114, 115.)

recessive: A genetic trait or disease that appears only in patients who have received two copies of a *mutant gene,* one from each parent.

reuptake: A process by which released *neurotransmitters* are absorbed for subsequent reuse.

ribonucleic acid: A chemical similar to a single strand of *DNA.* The sugar is ribose, not deoxyribose, hence RNA. In RNA, the letter U, which stands for uracil, is substituted for T in the genetic code. RNA delivers *DNA's* genetic message to the cytoplasm of a cell, where proteins are made.

serotonin: A *neurotransmitter* believed to play many roles, including, but not limited to, temperature regulation, sensory perception, and the onset of sleep. *Neurons* using serotonin as a transmitter are found in the brain and in the gut. A number of antidepressant drugs are targeted to brain serotonin systems.

spinal cord: The "other half" of the *central nervous system* (with the brain). The spinal cord is a cable that descends from the *brain stem* to the lower back. It consists of an inner core of *gray matter* surrounded by *white matter.* (See Figure 1, p. 110.)

stem cells: Undifferentiated cells that can grow into heart cells, kidney cells, or other cells of the body. Originally thought to be found only in embryos, stem cells in the brain have unexpectedly been discovered in adults. Researchers have shown on research animals that stem cells can be transplanted into various regions of the brain, where they develop into both *neurons* and *glia.*

sulcus: The shallower grooves on the brain's *cerebrum* (deeper grooves are called fissures). Plural is *sulci.*

synapse: The junction where an *axon* approaches another *neuron* or its extension (a *dendrite*); the point at which nerve-to-nerve communication occurs. Nerve impulses traveling down the *axon* reach the synapse and release *neurotransmitters* into the synaptic cleft, the tiny gap between *neurons.* (See Figures 5 and 6, pp. 138, 139.)

synaptic transmission: The process of cell-to-cell communication in the *central nervous system* (see Figures 5 and 6, pp. 114, 115), whereby one *neuron* sends a chemical signal across the synaptic cleft to another *neuron.*

temporal lobes: The parts of the *cerebrum* that are located on either side of the head, roughly beneath the temples in humans. These areas are involved in hearing, language, *memory* storage, and emotion. (See Figure 3, p. 112.)

thalamus: A brain structure located at the top of the *brain stem*, the thalamus acts as a two-way relay station, sorting, processing, and directing signals from the *spinal cord* and mid-brain structures to the *cerebrum*, and from the *cerebrum* down. (See Figure 2, p. 111.)

vestibular: Refers to the sense of balance. Many people with hearing loss also have some degree of balance difficulties, since the vestibular (or balance) system and the auditory (or hearing) systems are so closely related.

visual cortex: The area of the *cerebrum* that is specialized for vision. It lies primarily in the *occipital lobe* (see Figure 3, p. 112) at the rear of the brain, and is connected to the eyes by the optic nerves.

white matter: Brain or *spinal cord* tissue consisting primarily of the *myelin*-covered *axons* that extend from nerve cell bodies in the *gray matter* of the *central nervous system.*

SOURCES:

Stedman's Medical Dictionary, 24th Edition. Williams & Wilkins; Baltimore (1982).

Clayman C, ed. *The Human Body: An Illustrated Guide to Its Structure, Function, and Disorders.* Dorling Kindersley; New York (1995).

Posner MI, Raichle ME. *Images of Mind.* Scientific American Library; New York (1994).

Webster's New World Dictionary, 3rd College Edition. Simon & Schuster; New York (1991).

National Institute of Drug Abuse (NIDA). *Mind Over Matter Teachers Guide, Introduction and Background* (from the NIDA Web site).

National Human Genome Research Institute (NIH), www.nhgri.nih.gov.

Howard Hughes Medical Institute, *Blazing a Genetic Trail*, www.hhmi.org.

Society for Neuroscience. *Brain Facts, Fourth Edition.* Washington, DC (2002).

Marcus S, ed., *Neuroethics: Mapping the Field.* Dana Press; Washington, DC (2002).

Maps of the Brain

Figure 1

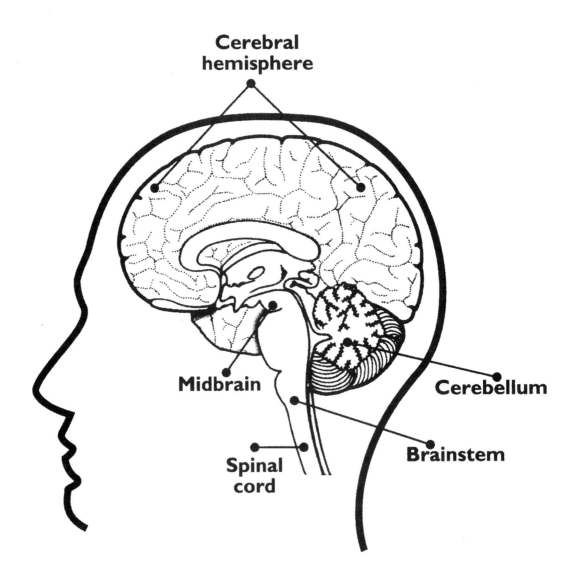

Figure 2

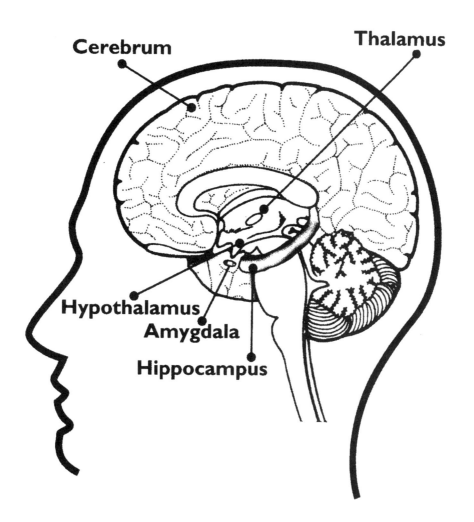

Figure 3

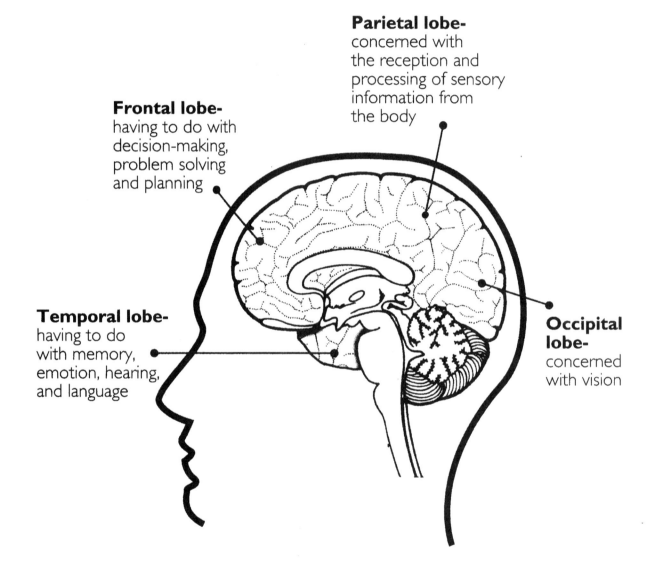

Parietal lobe-
concerned with
the reception and
processing of sensory
information from
the body

Frontal lobe-
having to do with
decision-making,
problem solving
and planning

Temporal lobe-
having to do
with memory,
emotion, hearing,
and language

**Occipital
lobe-**
concerned
with vision

Figure 4

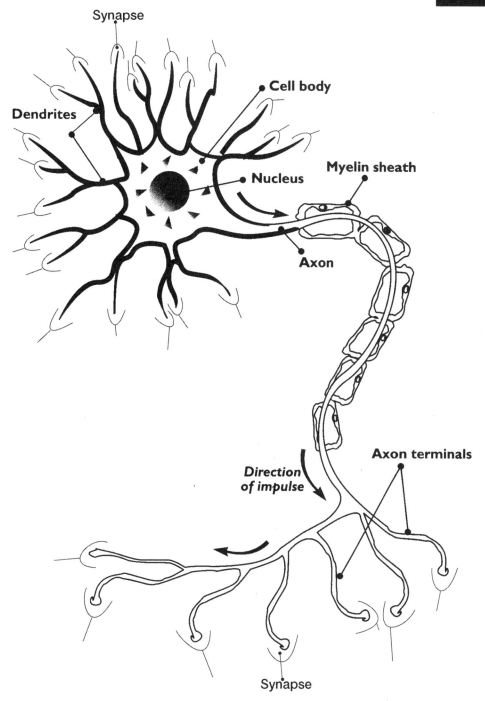

Figure 5

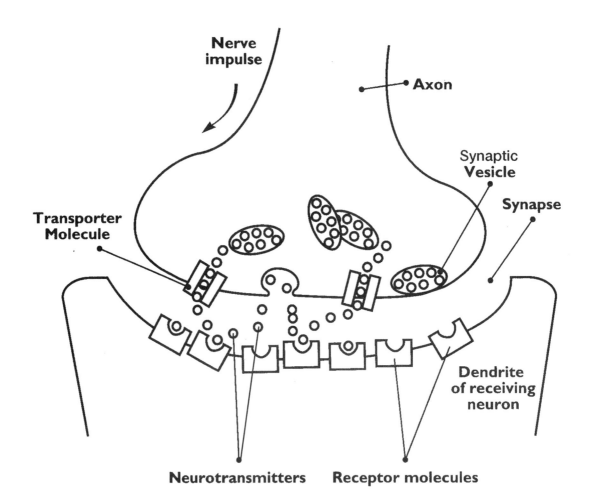

Nerve impulse

Axon

Synaptic **Vesicle**

Synapse

Transporter Molecule

Dendrite of receiving neuron

Neurotransmitters

Receptor molecules

Figure 6

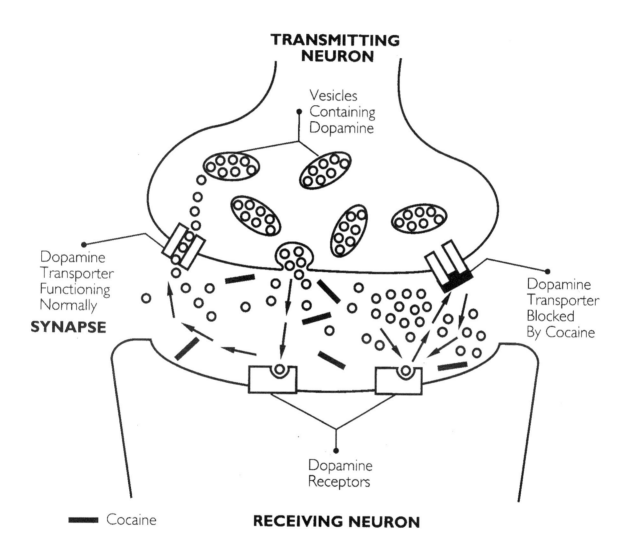

Resources on the Web

■ **GENERAL INFORMATION/SUPPORT**

American Academy of Neurology
www.aan.com

American Association of Suicidology
www.suicidology.org

American Psychiatric Association
www.psych.org

American Psychological Association
www.apa.org

Easter Seals
www.easterseals.com

Federation of Families for Children's Mental Health
www.ffcmh.org

Genetic Alliance
www.geneticalliance.org

Harvard Brain Tissue Resource Center
www.brainbank.mclean.org

NAMI (National Alliance on Mental Illness)
www.nami.org

NARSAD: The Mental Health Research Association
www.narsad.org

National Coalition of Creative Arts Therapies Associations (NCCATA)
www.nccata.org

National Mental Health Association
www.nmha.org

■ **FAMILY ASSISTANCE RESOURCES**

American Health Assistance Foundation
www.ahaf.org

Children of Aging Parents
www.caps4caregivers.org

Eldercare Locator
www.eldercare.gov

Family Caregiver Alliance
www.caregiver.org

Well Spouse Association
www.wellspouse.org

■ **GOVERNMENT RESOURCES**

Anxiety Disorders Education Program Library (NIH)
www.nimh.nih.gov

Centers for Disease Control and Prevention (CDC)
www.cdc.gov

National Cancer Institute (NIH)
www.cancer.gov

National Center for Complementary and Alternative Medicine (NIH)
www.nccam.nih.gov

National Eye Institute (NIH)
www.nei.nih.gov

National Heart, Lung, and Blood Institute (NIH)
www.nhlbi.nih.gov

National Institute on Aging (NIH)
www.nih.gov/nia

National Institute on Alcohol Abuse and Alcoholism (NIH)
www.niaaa.nih.gov

National Institute of Allergy and Infectious Diseases (NIH)
www.niaid.nih.gov

National Institute of Child Health and Human Development (NIH)
www.nichd.nih.gov

National Institute on Deafness and Other Communication Disorders (NIH)
www.nidcd.nih.gov

National Institute on Drug Abuse/NIDA (NIH)
www.nida.nih.gov

National Institute of Environmental Health Sciences (NIH)
www.niehs.nih.gov

National Institute of Mental Health (NIH)
www.nimh.nih.gov

National Institute of Neurological Disorders and Stroke/NINDS (NIH)
www.ninds.nih.gov

Office of Rare Diseases (NIH)
http://rarediseases.info.nih.gov

■ INFORMATION FOR ADULTS 50-PLUS

AARP
www.aarp.org

NRTA: *AARP's Educator Community*
www.aarp.org/nrta

National Institute on Aging (NIH)
(See p. 116.)

■ ACOUSTIC NEUROMA

Acoustic Neuroma Association
www.anausa.org

■ AGENESIS CORPUS CALLOSUM

The ACC Network
E-mail: um-acc@maine.edu

■ AGING-RELATED DISEASES

Alliance for Aging Research
www.agingresearch.org

National Council on Aging
www.ncoa.org

National Institute on Aging (NIH)
(See p. 116.)

Family Caregiver Alliance
(See p. 116.)

Children of Aging Parents
(See p. 116.)

Eldercare Locator
(See p. 116.)

■ AIDS DEMENTIA

CDC National Prevention Information Network
www.cdcnpin.org

Gay Men's Health Crisis (GMHC)
www.gmhc.org

National Institute of Allergy and Infectious Diseases (NIH)
(See p. 116.)

■ ALCOHOL AND DRUG ABUSE (Also see: Drug Abuse)

Al-Anon Family Groups Headquarters, Inc.
www.al-anon.alateen.org

Alcoholics Anonymous
www.alcoholics-anonymous.org

American Society of Addiction Medicine
www.asam.org

Betty Ford Center at Eisenhower
www.bettyfordcenter.org

National Clearinghouse for Alcohol & Drug Abuse Information
www.health.org

National Council on Alcoholism and Drug Dependence (NCADD)
www.ncadd.org

Recovery, Inc.
www.recovery-inc.org

National Institute on Alcohol Abuse and Alcoholism (NIH)
(See p. 116.)

■ ALZHEIMER'S DISEASE

Alzheimer's Association
www.alz.org

Alzheimer's Disease Education and Referral (ADEAR) Center/National Institute on Aging
www.alzheimers.org

Alzheimer's Research Forum
www.alzforum.org

Family Caregiver Alliance
(See p. 116.)

Children of Aging Parents
(See p. 116.)

■ AMYOTROPHIC LATERAL SCLEROSIS (ALS or Lou Gehrig's Disease)

The ALS Association
www.alsa.org

Les Turner ALS Foundation
www.lesturnerals.org

Muscular Dystrophy Association
(See p. 122.)

■ ANGELMAN SYNDROME (See: Rare Disorders)

■ ANOREXIA/BULIMIA (See: Eating Disorders)

■ ANXIETY DISORDERS

Anxiety Disorder Education Program Library
www.nimh.nih.gov

Freedom From Fear
www.freedomfromfear.org

National Anxiety Foundation
www.lexington-on-line.com/naf.html

■ APHASIA

National Aphasia Association
www.aphasia.org

■ ATAXIA AND ATAXIA-TELANGIECTASIA

A-T Children's Project
www.atcp.org

National Ataxia Foundation
www.ataxia.org

■ ATTENTION DEFICIT/HYPERACTIVITY DISORDER (ADHD) (See also: Learning Disabilities)

Attention Deficit Disorder Association
www.add.org

Children and Adults With Attention Deficit/Hyperactivity Disorder
www.chadd.org

■ AUTISM

Autism Genetic Resource Exchange
www.agre.org

Autism Society of America
www.autism-society.org

Autism Speaks
www.autismspeaks.org

Cure Autism Now Foundation
www.cureautismnow.org

National Alliance for Autism Research
www.naar.org

■ AUTOIMMUNE DISEASES (See: Neuroimmunological Disorders)

■ BACK PAIN (See: Pain, Chronic; Spine-Related Injury)

■ BATTEN DISEASE

Batten Disease Support and Research Association
www.bdsra.org

■ BEHAVIOR THERAPY

Association for Advancement of Behavior Therapy
www.aabt.org

■ **BEHCET'S DISEASE**

American Behcet's Disease Association
www.behcets.com

■ **BENIGN ESSENTIAL BLEPHAROSPASM**

Benign Essential Blepharospasm Research Foundation
www.blepharospasm.org

■ **BIRTH DEFECTS**

Birth Defect Research for Children
www.birthdefects.org

March of Dimes Birth Defects Foundation
www.marchofdimes.com

National Center on Birth Defects and Developmental Disabilities (CDC)
www.cdc.gov/ncbddd/bdlist.htm

■ **BLINDNESS/VISION IMPAIRMENT**

Helen Keller National Center for Deaf/Blind Youth and Adults
www.hknc.org

Lighthouse International
www.lighthouse.org

Prevent Blindness America
www.preventblindness.org

Research to Prevent Blindness
www.rpbusa.org

National Eye Institute (NIH)
(See p. 116.)

■ **BORDERLINE PERSONALITY DISORDER**

BPD Resource Center
www.bpdresourcecenter.org

Treatment and Research Advancements Association for Personality Disorders (TARA/APD)
www.tara4bpd.org

■ **BRAIN INJURY/PREVENTION**

Brain Injury Association of America
www.biausa.org

Brain Injury Services
www.braininjurysvcs.org

National Institute of Neurological Disorders and Stroke/NINDS (NIH)
www.ninds.nih.gov

Head Injury Hotline
www.headinjury.com

ThinkFirst Foundation
www.thinkfirst.org

■ **BRAIN TUMOR (See also: Pediatric Brain Tumor; Pituitary Disorders)**

American Brain Tumor Association
www.abta.org

Brain Tumor Society
www.tbts.org

Dana-Farber Cancer Institute
www.dana-farber.org

The Healing Exchange BRAIN TRUST
www.braintrust.org

National Brain Tumor Foundation
www.braintumor.org

■ **CEREBRAL PALSY**

United Cerebral Palsy/United Cerebral Palsy Research and Education Foundation
www.ucp.org

■ **CHARCOT-MARIE-TOOTH DISEASE**

Charcot-Marie-Tooth Association
www.charcot-marie-tooth.org

Muscular Dystrophy Association
(See p. 122.)

■ **CHIARI MALFORMATION (See: Spina Bifida; Syringomyelia)**

■ **COMA (See also: Brain Injury/Prevention)**

Coma Recovery Association
www.comarecovery.org

■ CONCUSSION (See: Brain Injury/
Prevention)

■ DEAFNESS/HEARING LOSS

**Alexander Graham Bell Association for the
Deaf and Hard of Hearing**
www.agbell.org

American Society for Deaf Children
www.deafchildren.org

Better Hearing Institute
www.betterhearing.org

**Self Help for Hard of Hearing
People/Cochlear Implant Division**
http://hearingloss.org/html/contact_us.html

**Laurent Clerc National Deaf Education Center
at Gallaudet University**
http://clerccenter.gallaudet.edu

National Cued Speech Association
www.cuedspeech.org

Self Help for Hard of Hearing People
www.shhh.org

■ DEJERINE-SOTTAS DISEASE

Muscular Dystrophy Association
(See p. 122.)

■ DEPRESSION/MANIC DEPRESSION

Depression and Bi-Polar Support Alliance
www.dbsalliance.org

**Depression and Related Affective Disorders
Association (DRADA)**
www.drada.org

**NARSAD: The Mental Health Research
Association**
www.narsad.org

National Institute of Mental Health (NIH)
(See p. 117.)

■ DIABETIC NEUROPATHY

The Neuropathy Association
www.neuropathy.org

**National Institute of Neurological Disorders
and Stroke/NINDS (NIH)**
www.ninds.nih.gov

■ DISABILITY AND REHABILITATION

Disabled Sports USA
www.dsusa.org

**The George Washington University HEATH
Resource Center**
www.heath.gwu.edu

Goodwill Industries International
www.goodwill.org

**National Dissemination Center for Children
With Disabilities**
www.nichcy.org

■ DIZZINESS (See: Vestibular Disorders)

■ DOWN SYNDROME

National Down Syndrome Society
www.ndss.org

■ DRUG ABUSE (See also: Alcohol and Drug
Abuse)

Do It Now Foundation
www.doitnow.org

National Families in Action
www.nationalfamilies.org

National Institute on Drug Abuse/NIDA (NIH)
(See p. 117.)

■ DYSAUTONOMIA

The Dysautonomia Foundation
www.familialdysautonomia.org

■ DYSLEXIA (See also: Learning Disabilities)

The International Dyslexia Association
www.interdys.org

■ DYSTONIA

Dystonia Medical Research Foundation
www.dystonia-foundation.org

■ **EATING DISORDERS**

National Association of Anorexia Nervosa and Associated Disorders
www.anad.org

National Eating Disorders Association
www.nationaleatingdisorders.org

■ **ENCEPHALITIS, RASMUSSEN'S (See: Neuroimmunological Disorders)**

■ **EPILEPSY**

Epilepsy Foundation
www.efa.org

■ **ESSENTIAL TREMOR/FAMILIAL TREMOR**

International Essential Tremor Foundation
www.essentialtremor.org

■ **FETAL ALCOHOL SYNDROME**

National Organization on Fetal Alcohol Syndrome
www.nofas.org

National Institute of Child Health and Human Development (NIH)
(See p. 117.)

National Institute on Alcohol Abuse and Alcoholism (NIH)
(See p. 116.)

■ **FRAGILE X SYNDROME**

FRAXA Research Foundation
www.fraxa.org

■ **FRIEDREICH'S ATAXIA**

Muscular Dystrophy Association
(See p. 122.)

■ **GAUCHER'S DISEASE**

National Gaucher Foundation
www.gaucherdisease.org

■ **GUILLAIN-BARRE SYNDROME**

GBS/CIDP Foundation International
www.gbsfi.com

■ **HEADACHE**

American Council for Headache Education/American Headache Society
www.achenet.org

Association for Applied Psychophysiology and Biofeedback
www.aapb.org

National Headache Foundation
www.headaches.org

■ **HEAD INJURY/TRAUMA (See: Brain Injury/Prevention; Coma)**

■ **HUNTINGTON'S DISEASE**

Hereditary Disease Foundation
www.hdfoundation.org

Huntington's Disease Society of America
www.hdsa.org

■ **HYDROCEPHALUS**

Guardians of Hydrocephalus Research Foundation
http://ghrf.homestead.com/ghrf.html

Hydrocephalus Association
www.hydroassoc.org

National Hydrocephalus Foundation
www.nhfonline.org

■ **JOSEPH DISEASES (See: Rare Disorders)**

■ **JOUBERT SYNDROME**

Joubert Syndrome Foundation
www.joubertsyndrome.org

■ **LEARNING DISABILITIES**

Learning Disabilities Association of America
www.ldaamerica.org

National Center for Learning Disabilities
www.ld.org

The International Dyslexia Association
(See p. 120.)

■ **LEIGH'S DISEASE (See: Rare Disorders)**

- **LEUKODYSTROPHY**

  United Leukodystrophy Foundation
  www.ulf.org

- **LOWE SYNDROME**

  Lowe Syndrome Association
  www.lowesyndrome.org

- **LUPUS**

  Lupus Foundation of America
  www.lupus.org

- **MACHADO-JOSEPH DISEASES (See: Rare Disorders)**

- **MEIGE SYNDROME (See: Benign Essential Blepharospasm)**

- **MENTAL RETARDATION**

  The Arc of the United States
  www.thearc.org

- **MOEBIUS SYNDROME (See: Rare Disorders)**

- **MULTIPLE SCLEROSIS**

  Multiple Sclerosis Association of America
  www.msaa.com

  Multiple Sclerosis Foundation
  www.msfocus.org

  National Multiple Sclerosis Society
  www.nmss.org

- **MUSCULAR DYSTROPHY**

  Muscular Dystrophy Association
  www.mdausa.org

- **MYASTHENIA GRAVIS**

  Myasthenia Gravis Foundation of America, Inc.
  www.myasthenia.org

  Muscular Dystrophy Association
  (See p. 122.)

- **MYOSITIS**

  The Myositis Association
  www.myositis.org

- **NARCOLEPSY (See also: Sleep Disorders)**

  Narcolepsy Network
  www.narcolepsynetwork.org

- **NEIMANN-PICK DISEASE (See: Rare Disorders)**

- **NEUROFIBROMATOSIS**

  Children's Tumor Foundation
  www.ctf.org

  Neurofibromatosis, Inc.
  www.nfinc.org

- **NEUROIMMUNOLOGICAL DISORDERS (See also: Multiple Sclerosis; Myasthenia Gravis)**

  American Autoimmune Related Diseases Association
  www.aarda.org

  Institute for Brain and Immune Disorders
  www.mmrf.org/research/brain_immune_disorder

  National Institute of Allergy and Infectious Diseases (NIH)
  (See p. 116.)

  National Institute of Environmental Health Sciences (NIH)
  (See p. 117.)

- **NEUROMUSCULAR DISEASES (See: Polio/Post-Polio Syndrome; Charcot-Marie-Tooth Disease)**

- **NEUROVASCULAR DISEASES (See: Stroke; Epilepsy; Brain Tumor)**

- **OBSESSIVE-COMPULSIVE DISORDER (OCD)**

  Obsessive-Compulsive Foundation
  www.ocfoundation.org

Trichotillomania Learning Center
www.trich.org

■ PAIN (CHRONIC) (See also: Spine-Related Injury/Back Pain)

American Chronic Pain Association
www.theacpa.org

American Pain Foundation
www.painfoundation.org

National Chronic Pain Outreach Association
www.chronicpain.org

■ PANIC DISORDERS (See: Anxiety Disorders)

■ PARALYSIS (See: Disability and Rehabilitation; Spinal Cord Injury)

■ PARKINSON'S DISEASE

American Parkinson Disease Association
www.apdaparkinson.org

Parkinson's Action Network
www.parkinsonsaction.org

The Parkinson's Disease Foundation
www.pdf.org

The Parkinson's Institute
www.thepi.org

■ PEDIATRIC BRAIN TUMOR (See also: Brain Tumor)

Brain Tumor Foundation for Children
www.braintumorkids.org

The Childhood Brain Tumor Foundation
www.childhoodbraintumor.org

Children's Brain Tumor Foundation
www.cbtf.org

Pediatric Brain Tumor Foundation
www.pbtfus.org

■ PEDIATRIC STROKE (See also: Stroke; Epilepsy; Cerebral Palsy)

Pediatric Stroke Network
www.pediatricstrokenetwork.com

■ PITUITARY DISORDERS (See also: Brain Tumor)

Pituitary Network Association
www.pituitary.org

■ POLIO/POST-POLIO SYNDROME

Post-Polio Health International
www.post-polio.org

■ POSTPARTUM DEPRESSION

Postpartum Support International
www.postpartum.net

■ POST-TRAUMATIC STRESS DISORDER

National Center for Post-Traumatic Stress Disorder
www.ncptsd.org

■ PRADER-WILLI SYNDROME

Prader-Willi Syndrome Association USA
www.pwsausa.org

■ PROGRESSIVE SUPRANUCLEAR PALSY

Society for Progressive Supranuclear Palsy
www.psp.org

■ PSEUDOTUMOR CEREBRI (See: Rare Disorders)

■ RARE DISORDERS

National Organization for Rare Disorders (NORD)
www.rarediseases.org

Office of Rare Diseases/National Institutes of Health (NIH)
(See p. 117.)

■ REFLEX SYMPATHETIC DYSTROPHY SYNDROME

RSDS Association
www.rsds.org

■ **RESTLESS LEGS SYNDROME**

RLS Foundation
www.rls.org

■ **RETT SYNDROME**

International Rett Syndrome Association
www.rettsyndrome.org

■ **REYE'S SYNDROME**

National Reye's Syndrome Foundation
www.reyessyndrome.org

■ **SCHIZOPHRENIA**

NAMI (National Alliance on Mental Illness)
www.nami.org

NARSAD: The Mental Health Research
Association
www.narsad.org

■ **SHY-DRAGER SYNDROME**

American Academy of Neurology
www.aan.com

■ **SJOGREN'S SYNDROME**

Sjogren's Syndrome Foundation
www.sjogrens.org

■ **SLEEP DISORDERS (See also: Narcolepsy)**

American Sleep Apnea Association
www.sleepapnea.org

National Sleep Foundation
www.sleepfoundation.org

■ **SMELL AND TASTE (Chemosensory) Disorders**

National Institute on Deafness and Other
Communication Disorders/NIDCD (NIH)
(See p. 117.)

■ **SOTOS SYNDROME**

Sotos Syndrome Support Association
www.well.com/user/sssa/

■ **SPASMODIC DYSPHONIA**

National Spasmodic Dysphonia Association
www.dysphonia.org

■ **SPASMODIC TORTICOLLIS**

National Spasmodic Torticollis Association
www.torticollis.org

■ **SPINA BIFIDA**

Spina Bifida Association of America
www.sbaa.org

■ **SPINAL CORD INJURY (See also: Disability and Rehabilitation)**

National Spinal Cord Injury Association
www.spinalcord.org

Paralyzed Veterans of America
www.pva.org

Spinal Cord Injury Network International
www.spinalcordinjury.org

■ **SPINAL MUSCULAR ATROPHY**

Families of Spinal Muscular Atrophy
www.curesma.org

■ **SPINE-RELATED INJURY/BACK PAIN (See also: Pain [Chronic])**

North American Spine Society
www.spine.org

■ **STROKE**

American Stroke Association
www.strokeassociation.org

National Stroke Association
www.stroke.org

■ **STURGE-WEBER DISEASE**

The Sturge-Weber Foundation
www.sturge-weber.com

■ **STUTTERING**

National Stuttering Association
www.westutter.org

Stuttering Foundation of America
www.stutteringhelp.org

■ SYRINGOMYELIA

American Syringomyelia Alliance Project
www.asap.org

■ TARDIVE DYSKINESIA/TARDIVE DYSTONIA

National Institute of Neurological Disorders
and Stroke/NINDS (NIH)
www.ninds.nih.gov

■ TAY-SACHS DISEASE

National Tay-Sachs and Allied Diseases
Association
www.ntsad.org

■ TINNITUS

American Tinnitus Association
www.ata.org

■ TOURETTE SYNDROME

Tourette Syndrome Association
www.tsa-usa.org

■ TRIGEMINAL NEURALGIA

Trigeminal Neuralgia Association
www.endthepain.org

■ TUBEROUS SCLEROSIS

National Tuberous Sclerosis Association
www.tsalliance.org

■ VESTIBULAR DISORDERS

Vestibular Disorders Association
www.vestibular.org

■ VON HIPPEL-LINDAU SYNDROME

Von Hippel-Lindau (VHL) Syndrome
Family Alliance
www.vhl.org

■ WILLIAMS SYNDROME

Williams Syndrome Association
www.williams-syndrome.org

■ WILSON'S DISEASE

Wilson's Disease Association International
www.wilsonsdisease.org

■ FOR FURTHER INFORMATION

These organizations focus primarily on research, professional support, and/or advocacy. They may, however, be able to provide information or assistance to the public on a limited basis.

American Academy of Anti-Aging Medicine
www.worldhealth.net

American Academy of Child and Adolescent Psychiatry
www.aacap.org

American Academy of Pediatrics
www.aap.org

American Association for Geriatric Psychiatry
www.aagponline.org

American College of Medical Genetics
www.acmg.net

American College of Mental Health Administration
www.acmha.org

American College of Neuropsychopharmacology
www.acnp.org

American Managed Behavioral Healthcare Association
www.ambha.org

American Occupational Therapy Association
www.aota.org

American Society of Neuroradiology
www.asnr.org

Coordinated Campaign for Learning Disabilities
www.ldonline.org/ccldinfo

The Gerontological Society of America
www.geron.org

Judge David L. Bazelon Center for Mental Health Law
www.bazelon.org

Mental Illness Research Association
www.miraresearch.org

National Organization on Disability
www.nod.org

Pilot International Foundation
www.pilotinternational.org

Society of Toxicology
www.toxicology.org

ZERO TO THREE
www.zerotothree.org

Acknowledgments

The Dana Sourcebook of Brain Science
Resources for Teachers and Students
Fourth Edition

David Balog, Editor

Contributors:
Lynn Wecker, Ph.D., University of South Florida College of Medicine,
    Scientific Consultant
Gerard Teachman, Ph.D., Mental Illness Research Association,
    Education Advisor
David Alpay, University of Toronto, Student Assistant
Kevin Long, Ph.D., Chemicon International and University of California,
    San Diego Extension, Scientific Contributor
Brenda Patoine, Contributing Writer
Uri Treisman, Ph.D., Charles A. Dana Center,
    University of Texas, Austin, Editorial Advisor

DANA
PRESS

Jane Nevins, Editor in Chief, Dana Press
Cynthia A. Read, Associate Director, Dana Press
Kristine Pauls, Production Editor, Dana Press

Credits:

5–7: Dana Alliance for Brain Initiatives

9: University of Maryland

11: *top to bottom*, Marcus E. Raichle, M.D., Washington University School of Medicine, St. Louis, Department of Radiology and Neurology; University of Arizona Board of Regents; Peter Melzer, Vanderbilt Kennedy Center for Research in Human Development

12: Dana Press

14: Randy Blakely and Sally Shroeter, Vanderbilt Center for Molecular Neuroscience

20–21: Eileen Whalen, except for neuron artwork on p. 21 provided by National Institute on Drug Abuse

23: Dana Alliance for Brain Initiatives

25–46: Dana Alliance for Brain Initiatives and Dana Press

48: University of Pennsylvania Department of Neuroscience

51: Max-Planck Institute *(top)*; Cold Spring Harbor Laboratory *(bottom)*

53: University of Bristol, *(l)*; J. Rehg/Zuma Images, *(r)*

69: *clockwise, from top, left*, W.H. Freeman, W.H. Freeman, Knopf, Simon & Schuster

70: *clockwise, from top, left*, Viking Adult, John Wiley & Sons, Inc., and Dana Press, MIT Press, Viking Adult

78: *clockwise, from top, left*, Penguin Classics, Vintage, Scribner, Dial Press, HarcourtBrace

80: *clockwise, from top, left*, Vintage, Doubleday, Franklin Watts, Vintage

81: *(l-r)*, Vintage, Carroll & Graf

83–84, 88: Max Taylor Photography

94: Elaine Snell, European Dana Alliance for the Brain

110–115: National Institute on Drug Abuse

Cover design, Kristine Pauls

Text design, William Bragg

Index

communicating with the public
 about stem cells, 23
 as vision and commitment of Dana Alliance for
  Brain Initiatives, 47, 48, 49
computed tomography (CT or CAT scan), 29, 36,
 56–57, 101
concussions, multiple, 58
conditioning, 44–45, 57–58
Conlan, Roberta, 97
consciousness, definition of, 101
coordination, 57–58
cortex, Classroom DVD lesson on, 56–57. *See also*
 specific parts of the cortex
corticotropin-releasing factor, 40
cortisol, 40–41, 59, 101
Creating Brain, The: Neuroscience of Genius
 (Andreasen), 94–95
creativity, nature and nurture of, 27–28. *See also* free
 will versus nature and past experiences
Crick, Francis, 19, 71
Curie, Marie, 6
Curious Incident of the Dog in the Night-Time, The
 (Haddon), 82
cystic fibrosis, genetic predisposition to, 21
Cytowic, Richard, 80

D

Damasio, Antonio, 12, 68, 75, 89–90
Damasio, Hannah, 89–90
Dana Alliance for Brain Initiatives
 commitment, bench to bedside, 49
 goals, 49–52
 great brain books, list of, 68–72
 online information about, 93
 scientists of the Dana Alliance, list of books
  written by, 72–77
 strategy for success, 52–53
 tools for achieving goals, 54–55
 vision and goals statement, 47–48
Dana Foundation, 94
Dana Guide to Brain Health, The (Bloom, Beal, and
 Kupfer, eds.), 76, 96
dana.org, 93, 94
Dana Press, 94
*Dana Sourcebook of Immunology, The: Resources for
 Secondary and Post-Secondary Teachers and
 Students* (Gordon, ed.), 97
da Vinci, Leonardo, 27
deafness, resources for help with, 120
decision and action, Shakespeare on, 88–90
declarative memory, 104
Dejerine–Sottas disease resource, 120
dementia, definition of, 101

dendrites, 101, 113, 114. *See also* axons and axonal
 guidance
deoxyribonucleic acid. *See* DNA
DePaulo, J. Raymond, Jr., 37–38, 77
dependence, definition of, 101, 108
depression
 Classroom DVD lesson on, 60–61
 definition of, 102
 genes and environmental factors, 6
 improving treatment for, 47, 50, 52
 manic-depressive illness, 37, 50, 120
 resources for help with, 120, 123
Depression and the Brain (Classroom DVD),
 60–61
Descartes, René, 12
*Descartes' Error: Emotion, Reason, and the Human
 Brain* (Damasio), 12, 68
development stages of the brain, 14–16, 52
diabetic neuropathy resources, 120
Dickens, Charles, 79
disability and rehabilitation, resources for help
 with, 120
diseases and embryonic stem cells, 24. *See also*
 specific diseases
disorders. *See specific disorders*
disuse atrophy versus facilitation, 45–46
Diving Bell and the Butterfly, The (Bauby), 80
DNA: The Secret of Life (Watson), 74
DNA (deoxyribonucleic acid)
 definition of, 102
 double helix structure, 19, 102
 genome of, 103
 guide to, 20
 overview, 10
 role of, 16–17
 See also genes
DNA variation, mapping, 17
dominant (gene), 102
donor site of embolism, 36
dopamine, 50, 61–63, 102, 106
dopamine receptors, map showing, 115
dopamine transport blockers, 63–64
Dostoevsky, Fyodor, 79
double helix, 102
Down syndrome resource, 120
drug addiction
 Classroom DVD lessons on, 61–64
 narcotic drugs, 9, 105
 resources for help with, 120
 reversing changes to brain from, 47, 52
drug (pharmaceutical) discovery, expansion of, 55
drugs and the brain, Shakespeare on, 86–87
Drugs and the Brain (Snyder), 68–69
DVD. *See* Classroom DVD